THE PATH OF INTENTION

FIVE HABITS TO OPTIMIZE YOUR HEALTH
AND CREATE A LIFE YOU LOVE

The Path of Intention © Copyright 2022
Libby Wilson, M.D., and Nathan Long

For more information, email drlibby@bestlifefunctionalmedicine.com or natelong@longroadcrossfit.com.

ISBN: 979-8-9863363-0-5

THE PATH OF INTENTION

FIVE HABITS TO OPTIMIZE YOUR HEALTH
AND CREATE A LIFE YOU LOVE

LIBBY WILSON M.D.
&
NATHAN LONG

GET YOUR FREE
PATH PLAYBOOK!

To get the best experience with this book, download The Path Playbook. This guide helps you to implement our recommendations faster and take the next steps more seamlessly, so you can improve your health, happiness, and fulfillment.

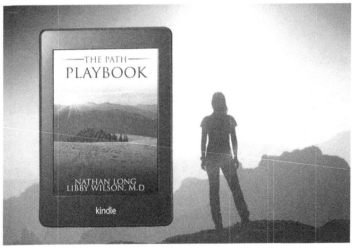

You can get a copy by visiting:
www.thepathofintention.com

TABLE OF CONTENTS

We dedicate this book to our spouses— Andy and Crystal. Thank you for being our biggest cheerleaders, best friends, and support system.

FOREWORD

WHY YOU SHOULD CARE

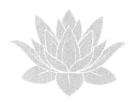

If you haven't been thinking about how you are aging now and you haven't been taking steps proactively to manage it, then by the time you finally address it, it may be too late. Aging is inevitable, but how you age—that, my friend—is within your control.

In terms of lifespan (how long you live) and healthspan (your number of active, healthy years), you have to be intentional by thinking about what you truly want for your life and making sure you are on a path that will get you there. If you don't know where you are going, any path will take you there. In terms of aging, this means chronic disease, decreased bone and muscle mass, and the dependence on others to care for you. You have to pause, determine your desired destination, and make sure you are headed on the right path forward.

The solution to this problem that we all face is prioritizing our health and being intentional. You'll hear this concept of intentionality come up repeatedly in this book. There are two paths—the autopilot default path and the path of intention. The autopilot path is what happens automatically, without forethought and planning. We recommend the path of intention with a purposeful, desired destination. This is challenging amidst our busy lives with so many things vying for our time and attention. Like paying into a retirement account, the sooner you start, the better off you are. It's never too late to start though. Small lifestyle hacks deposited daily over time build up to yield huge results.

The way you create an extended lifespan and healthspan is by intentionally incorporating the five factors of health into your daily life. The core of this book is about these five factors—sleep, diet, exercise, relationships, and mindset. We'll examine each of these factors deeply, show you how to determine where you are, and give you actionable steps to implement now to move you further down your desired path.

This book is more than a book about health. We want to show you not just how to have amazing health and longevity but also how to create a life you truly love now. For a fulfilling life, you want to be on a path of intention too. It's important to make sure you aren't delaying happiness till later. Tomorrow isn't guaranteed. Create a life for yourself NOW that is full of health and vibrancy and that fulfills your life's passion. You can have your cake and eat it too with intentionality, planning, and small, consistent daily actions repeated over time. In the beginning, you won't notice much change, but over time the results are extraordinary. Don't confuse simple with easy. The steps aren't complicated, but to have an amazing, abundant life the steps have to be purposeful and consistent. We are going to show you how. Are you ready? Let's go.

INTRODUCTION

FOUR PATHS

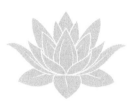

LIBBY'S PATH

I was a family practitioner for 20 years. I went to medical school with hopes and dreams of helping people become the healthiest version of themselves. That's what doctors do, right? I was hardworking, smart, and naive. I hustled in high school to get good grades to prepare for college. I hustled in college to get into medical school. The hustle continued in medical school to get the M.D.—to finally complete my education, establish a practice, and live out my lifelong dream of helping people be healthy. It was disappointing to realize after 11 years of higher education and a large student loan debt, that things weren't what I thought they were going to be.

Conventional medicine is appropriate for sick care. If you have strep throat, a broken leg, or heart disease, I

| 5

highly recommend you see a conventional medical doctor. Conventional medicine, which I trained in and practiced for all those years, is good at sick care but, in my opinion, not so good at healthcare. Thirty patients per day, 15 minutes per patient, with much of the visit centered around what the insurance company needs to be documented to pay for the visit. This model didn't allow me time to focus on what was truly important to the patient and certainly didn't leave much time for health optimization either.

I felt trapped and didn't know how to change my life, and I certainly had no idea how to change the broken system that I was a part of.

For years, I prioritized health and fitness for myself, but it seemed like I was living in two different worlds. My personal world was my healthy life—before work at the gym and after work with my family. My work life looked much different. I prescribed pill after pill to put Band-Aids on the plethora of problems that patients presented to me each day. While this method was helping their symptoms and improving their lab results, I wasn't really making them healthier or better off in the long run. I lacked fulfillment because I knew deep down inside, I really wasn't making a difference.

One day, at the 5:30 a.m. CrossFit class at Long Road CrossFit in Urbana, Ohio, I noticed a poster from Ben Bergeron titled "The 5 Factors of Health." Apparently, Nate Long had recently hung it up right in the middle of the gym. I noticed it immediately. The poster stated that the keys to health were diet, exercise, sleep, mindset, and relationships. "YES!" I screamed silently inside my head. "This is what I should be focusing on with my patients when I get to work in a couple of hours." However, in the constraints of my current practice model, I recognized that wasn't how my day was going to play out. A seed was planted though. I knew at that moment there had to be another way.

There are moments in our lives that change us. Moments after which we are never the same. That was one of those moments for me. I didn't yet know how, but I knew I was going to figure out a better way to fulfill the passion that was sparked inside of me years before when I decided to go to medical school.

Several months later, I signed up for a continuing education class in functional medicine. I had never heard of functional medicine during my conventional medical education. I learned, in that first course, that functional medicine aims to get to the root cause of symptoms patients present with, instead of just treating the symptoms. It seeks to fix imbalances before overt disease develops. Its focus is to accomplish this as naturally as possible with a combination of herbs, supplements, and lifestyle medicine. And guess what— like CrossFit, functional medicine ascribes to the same five modifiable lifestyle factors that are the keys to optimal health: diet, exercise, sleep, mindset, and relationships.

Isn't it interesting how things work out? My hobby, CrossFit, was now intersecting with my new career path, functional medicine. When your passion becomes your career, it no longer seems like work, so it didn't take long to learn functional medicine, figure out a way to do things differently, and create my own dream practice. Now I feel like I'm truly living my American Dream.

When Nate approached me about an idea he had for a book, I was all in. We always have choices in life—stay the same, or do something. I am grateful to Nate and CrossFit for giving me the push to do something. In the gym he encourages me to lift heavier weights or go faster. Now he is pushing me to get moving on a dream we both have in common— writing a book to share our knowledge and inspire others to live their healthiest, best, and most fulfilling life.

Now, in addition to being a board-certified family practitioner, I am also a functional medicine practitioner certified by The Institute of Functional Medicine and the Kalish Institute. Additionally, I am L1 CrossFit-certified and a Life and Weight Loss coach. I left my thriving family practice behind to open my dream business, Best Life Functional Medicine, where I work with health-conscious people who have been trying their best to take care of themselves but, despite their effort, haven't been seeing the results they are hoping for, that is, until they come and we work together. I also work with patients who aren't finding answers to their problems in conventional medicine.

NATE'S PATH

WHILE LIBBY MAY HAVE HAD THE VISION OF WHAT SHE WAS GOING to be at a pretty early stage of her life, it could not have been more different for me. My father was a junior high school teacher and coach with the discipline of a drill sergeant. My parents separated when I was a toddler, and my dad went on to remarry a few years later to the most selfless, amazing woman I have ever met. My stepmom worked her way up in the corporate world with nothing more than an amazing work ethic and an unwillingness to waiver from who she was. While their marriage was not a model of what I wanted mine to be when I grew up, they taught me some codes to live by that mirror *Cowboy Ethics* by James P. Owen. They taught me how to always be true to who I am and live with courage; to give 100 percent, no matter what job I am doing; that there is only one way to do something, the right way; that if you start something, you damn well better finish it; and that a "please" and a "thank you" can go a long way.

Why does all that matter? For me, a guy who never really had a clear picture of what he wanted to be when he grew up, it helped lay a foundation for a "successful" life. When you are willing to work hard and realize there is no such thing as failure, only an opportunity to learn and grow, then you go after your American Dream, even if you discover it at the age of 38.

As Libby stated, some moments change our lives forever. Mine was in year 12 of my teaching career. I heard the snarky and bleak comments, "Just livin' the dream" and "It is how it is," for the last time from the people that were supposed to be leading our school district. On my 38th birthday, in 2020, I put in my resignation and left behind the comfort of a state teacher retirement fund, job security, and great insurance.

Years earlier, my wife, Crystal, and I had found our love for CrossFit, health, and wellness. After a year at Practice CrossFit, Crystal and I decided that the CrossFit community we found in Troy, Ohio, was too good not to share in our local area. In 2013, we opened Long Road CrossFit in Urbana, Ohio, all while working our full-time jobs. What started as nothing more than a 10-member, 1,000-square-foot passion project, has grown into a two-location, 250-plus-member community of people that support one another in creating their American Dream and living their best life.

Whether it is coaching classes at the gym, running a business, or helping build teams, I've come to realize that my passion is helping others reach goals and push to their true potential. After attending Ben Bergeron's affiliate immersions program in 2018 at CrossFit New England, my life was changed forever. Listening and learning from Ben and his team in Boston helped give me a kickstart in my current life that has pushed me to new levels as a business owner, leader, friend, husband, and father.

I have come to realize that it is OK if your passion and interests change over time. How are you expected to choose a career at 18 that you are going to enjoy when you are 40? As people, we change, as do our interests and our goals. Just because we are told by society that we are supposed to pick a 30-year career to work hard at, whether we grow to hate it or not, is not actually how life has to be. Through CrossFit, reading hundreds of books, and being around amazing people like Libby, I've come to realize that the five factors in the chapters to come—sleep, diet, exercise, relationships, and mindset—will help us all lead a life of love and happiness. So do not worry, there is hope. You do not have to wait until you retire to have a life that you love.

OUR PATH

THIS BOOK IS A COLLABORATIVE EFFORT. NATE AND I SHARE A passion for helping others create optimal health and a fulfilling life. As already mentioned, the idea for the book was Nate's. He approached me one morning in August of 2021 with the idea for a book. The idea started by comparing a person's health to their retirement account. Small deposits in the retirement account make for a nice nest egg in the future and the sooner you start the easier it is. The same is true for your health.

We both believe that the keys to health, as you'll learn in the chapters that follow and that we've already mentioned, are the following five modifiable lifestyle factors: sleep, diet, exercise, mindset, and relationships. Small, consistent daily steps in those areas bring about changes and benefits to a person's healthspan and lifespan.

A month later, we met and brainstormed an outline and then started writing. We weren't sure how it would all fit together or who would do what initially. Over the next several months, as we worked on a shared document, it just flowed and fit nicely together.

My contribution was approaching each topic from a medical standpoint ("Dr. Libby's Tips") and Nate contributed the action plans ("Nate's Take"). Everything else is a combination of both of our voices working together to make things easy to understand, actionable, and enjoyable to read. As we wrapped up the rough draft, it became evident that we worked on this book in the same fashion as I work with patients in my functional medicine practice. After consulting with the patient and reviewing their labs, I design the plan and explain to them what is happening with them in terms of their health, why it is likely happening, and what steps we can take to fix it. Then my health coach helps the patient implement the plan. No plan works without implementation. The same is true in this book. As a doctor, I hope to help you understand the importance of each factor, and Nate, as a trainer and coach, shows how to take that information and put it into action.

Your Path

Prioritizing your health, by instituting some of the health hacks we provide in the following pages will not only help you feel great but give you the confidence that you are proactively extending your lifespan and your healthspan too. It really works. Here's the thing—small actions repeated over time create HUGE results. Intentionality is the KEY to success. It takes time to see the results. Most people give up way too soon. Don't be like most people.

I've seen this play out. I've had patients in their sixties who aren't healthy enough to attend their grandchildren's sporting events. I've had patients who are much too young plagued with crippling dementia, making them 100 percent dependent on the care of others. I've had patients who can't go anywhere that involves steps. I've had patients who can't get up if they fall. That was my old practice. Now I have a practice full of healthy patients. The patients I partner with now are proactive. We work together as a team to fix the underlying problems and create true health. Some of my current patients are in their seventies or eighties and are healthier than patients I've previously cared for in their forties. These patients are free of prescription meds and free of a life structured around the next doctor's appointment. They not only feel great, but they are thriving. They have choices because they aren't limited by sickness and poor health. What we are going to share in the pages that follow can work for anyone. It could work for my previous patients too. The only difference is none of this can be done for you. YOU need to control your destiny.

The sooner you start, the more you prioritize your health, the more freedom you'll create for yourself. This freedom, due to improved health, gets you out of survival mode, and all of a sudden you see opportunities that likely were there all along, but just not recognizable when your body and your mind were focused on staying alive. You begin to thrive, not just survive. I've seen it in myself. I've seen it in Nate, and I've seen it in countless patients. Don't wait. By the time you make the time, it may be too late. The most important thing to remember is that there is no one-size-fits-all method to finding true happiness. Much of what Nate and I learned over the years has been through trial and error. The good news is nothing is set in stone and everyone's path is going to look a little bit different. The most important thing of all is that we take action in making changes that lead us to a more fulfilling life.

Congratulations on taking the first step! You have the book, let's dive in and get started on making deposits into your health account, optimizing your healthspan, and moving YOU towards thriving not just surviving.

CHAPTER ONE

THE AMERICAN DREAM

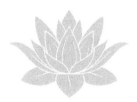

SUCCESS

I used to think the American Dream was available to us all if we worked hard and saved for retirement. THEN, one day, far into the future, after all that sacrifice and hard work, it would finally pay off. We could set the job aside and free up time to be happy and do the things we enjoy doing—in our sixties if all goes well. That was the old me. I now know that you don't have to wait to be happy. We can choose happiness along the journey and not just delay it until we get there, because here's the thing—there is no THERE to get to. We often think we'll be happy when (fill in the blank) happens only to learn that happiness is fleeting. Then we think we need a new goal, and we repeat the process again and again and again, all the while delaying the happiness that was a choice for us all along. Happiness is short term, but fulfillment is forever. How can we stop chasing the shiny things on the outside that we are told will bring us short-term "happiness" and start filling that void on the inside that helps bring fulfillment to our lives?

Every little kid, as they begin school, sets out to be successful. Right? In kindergarten, you strive to achieve the optimal placement on the behavior color chart, get a sticker on your paper from your teacher, and hopefully become student of the month. Kids learn from a very young age how to earn their worthiness. This is often achieved by complying, meeting expectations of others, and good ole hard work. I guess at age five, kids may not be thinking about this too much, but their parents sure are. Their little eyes are watching, and they are picking up the cues from those around them about what success looks like. They are unconsciously establishing their definition of success and developing their own belief system. But have you ever really stopped and thought about it? What *is* success anyway? What do we truly want for our kids, and ourselves, for that matter?

According to Google, success is **"the status of having achieved and accomplished an aim or objective."** Being successful means the achievement of desired visions and planned goals. Success is "attaining wealth, prosperity, and/or fame." When I read these definitions, I immediately think, "Ah, that's living the dream that so many speak of." What is the American Dream anyway, and where does that term, that's tossed around so commonly, even come from?

"JUST LIVIN' THE DREAM"

IN 1963, MARTIN LUTHER KING JR. GAVE THE "I HAVE A DREAM" speech at the Lincoln Memorial where he stood in front of thousands of Americans to protest the social injustice of African Americans. While at the time, Dr. King's primary focus was on equal rights and opportunities for all American citizens, the dream he spoke of would also provide EVERY citizen, no matter their race, religion, or creed, the same freedoms. These freedoms were transcribed by our founding fathers nearly 200 years prior in the Declaration of Independence. These were freedoms that guaranteed our right to life, liberty, and the pursuit of happiness. This was their dream, and we believe this was the foundation of the "American Dream." It is the ability for you to pursue happiness.

Fast forward 246 years. Walking into work on Monday, you pass Mike. Being the caring person you are, you greet him, "Good morning, Mike. How's it going?"

He lays on you the most overused line, "Just livin' the dream," with the thickest level of sarcastic tone.

How many times is this line used a day around the United States? How many times have you used it? This should be a wake-up call to all Americans. We have to look at ourselves and ask, what the hell has happened over the last 250 years that so many Americans are quoting that same line, with that same tone, EVERY SINGLE DAY?

BELIEFS

IN THE ABOVE EXAMPLE, MIKE AND MOST PEOPLE ARE JUST SAYING this, and they aren't really thinking about what they mean. But it's very important to pause and think about what we mean when we say that. Our version of the American Dream comes to us from our beliefs. Our beliefs are often created by our life experiences. We learned from our parents, who learned from their parents.

The unintentional beliefs handed down to us may be good, they may not be so good, but they are usually automatic. Beliefs are really nothing other than thoughts that we think again and again and again. We can decide if we want to keep thinking them, or we could decide to take action and change them. We could intentionally choose some different thoughts that may serve us better. These new thoughts repeated over time would create new beliefs, creating the life of OUR dreams.

With intentionality we can choose our thoughts, which create our beliefs regarding happiness, and create action steps to actually make those things happen. The only way to make a dream a reality is by action. Martin Luther King didn't just have a strong belief in a cause. He acted with lunch counter boycotts, bus boycotts, sit-ins, marches, voter registration campaigns, and peaceful protests of unjust laws. Dr. King was arrested 29 times for putting his words into action, and despite the setbacks, he never stopped pushing forward to pursue his dream. Like him, to create change you need to take action. Not just autopilot default action, but intentional action. Tony Robbins commented, "The only impossible journey is the one you never begin." While change can be scary, without action, your goals are nothing more than a dream.

WHERE ARE YOU AT?

WHAT DO YOU BELIEVE? WHY? IS YOUR PLAN CURRENTLY working for you, or is there something else, another way, that may work better? Is the path you set out on one that you created, or was it someone else's road map to happiness? If you think you may be driving your car in the wrong direction, it might be time to pull over and reassess your road map.

We were all handed down some default beliefs. It's just our choice whether we want to continue believing them and continue on this autopilot default path OR change them. This is the beginning of how we determine what the American Dream means to us, personally. This is how we begin to define our authentic, best life. Remember, we are in the driver's seat on our life's journey, so now we must determine the path we want to be on.

We all need to ask ourselves the first question, "Where am I at?"

CHAPTER TWO

BACK TO THE FUTURE

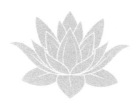

"Hey, Siri, take me to the future …"

If we were able to fast forward to get a glimpse of our future self like Marty McFly and Doc Brown did in *Back to the Future II*, would we actually want to see it? I suspect many of us would be peeking through our fingers like we were watching a scary movie, feeling a little unsure of what is going to be behind that door. If we understand where we want to go, plan intentionally, and execute that plan, pending any unforeseen events, we should have a pretty good idea of what we are going to be seeing, shouldn't we?

We believe if you took a survey of people across the United States of what their definition of success is, you would get a million different answers. However, within those million different answers, you could probably find some similarities. They probably all would include specifics about finances, career, health, and family. However, when asked how they plan to get to this life that is successful, we're not sure many would be able to list anything other than the prescription they have been told since grade school. They just get on the bus to success that starts in kindergarten, and hopefully they will be stepping off on easy street 50 years later as they approach retirement, ready to kick their feet up and start enjoying life.

Interestingly, in our early years of adulthood, our health is usually a given, barring any debilitating genetic issues or injuries. Our emphasis is on putting in the time to become established in a job or a career path that will allow us to be financially settled. But as time passes, a shift happens. The health that we could easily and without consequence take for granted is no longer a guarantee. As we become more financially secure, this is a great time to STOP and see if we are on the right path in all areas of our life. If we don't, we end up with the opposite of what we had in our early years. We no longer have to fight for financial and career success, but we have to fight to earn back our health. Most would trade money to have their health back at this point without question.

AUTOPILOT

Sara worked hard her whole life. She had a corporate job and—like everyone else—started at the bottom of the totem pole. She worked tirelessly. She did so much more than just show up and do her job. It didn't take long for others to recognize that she was a leader in her field. Over the years, she received promotions, and by her late thirties, she was the COO of a major corporation. Sara was living the dream. Her hard work was being noticed, and it paid off. The problem was, between work and family, Sara had no time to take care of herself or to prioritize her marriage. It didn't bother her too much because she was in good health and really didn't have any specific needs. Her husband knew she loved him and they would have time to reconnect later—when life slowed down. The years piled on and so did the weight.

Fast forward to age 65. Sara is ready to retire. Her marriage ended years earlier, but at least now she finally has the time to take care of herself. But now she worries if it is too late. She's 80 pounds overweight, her joints ache, and she struggles to get up off the ground. Her only son and his wife have struggled with fertility issues, but after many years of waiting, her first grandbaby is on the way. All of a sudden, Sara's health is a top priority. But is it too late? She's lived the American Dream, worked hard, and done all the right things to be a career success. She built a financially stable life. Medicare has kicked in, and she has saved enough to financially support herself without going to work. But her health, the health that she has always taken for granted, is no longer there. Happiness, over the years, has been a series of highs and lows. Now as life has slowed down and she has time to reflect, she is not sure if she has lived any kind of "dream."

Was Sara actually chasing her life's vision of what happiness is supposed to be? Was that the game plan she laid out for herself when she was in her late teenage years? Was it even a vision at all, or did she just follow a path that was set out for her? Heck, now that she thinks of it, how was she even supposed to know what she wanted to do for the rest of her life at 18?

She jumped into college, graduated, then luckily, jumped right into her career. It felt like she has been in fast forward ever since. She never took the time to stop and "smell the roses," to reflect on where she was in life and make adjustments where things were unbalanced. She was too busy doing all the things that each day demanded. Is that the way it is supposed to be? Put our blinders on, work hard, only to finally take them off and realize that we have been rowing our boat incredibly hard in the wrong direction over all of these years. It's at this point that it hits us—we have left our health and happiness in the wake of what we thought was fulfillment.

Instead, shouldn't we be striving for a level of self-actualization? Finding a path that gives us the most fulfillment and pushes our potential as humans. One that provides a life of experiences and pushes all of us "to become everything one is capable of becoming," according to Abraham Maslow. Maslow is an American psychologist who developed a hierarchy of needs to explain human motivation. They are, in this order: physiological needs, safety needs, love and belonging needs, esteem needs, and self-actualization needs. Sure, Sara successfully met her basic psychological and safety needs, but now she yearns for more and worries she doesn't have the health and years left to achieve it.

There is a different way. We have choices.

We could choose to make life decisions based on chasing nirvana, an ideal place of perfect happiness, rather than chasing a good pension and medical benefits. We could choose to make decisions based on what is morally right, instead of financially right. We could create a list of core values that resonate with our innermost self and let those guide our journey through life. We could choose to create our own path through exploration rather than follow the cookie-cutter path of happiness that society has laid out in front of us.

We believe there is a path that everyone can take and that will not prioritize our immediate financial needs before our long-term health and wellness needs. There is a balance we can reach in life that not only provides us the stability of our basic sociological needs, but also allows us to enjoy the journey for which life is. With this balance we do not have to live in a state of fast forward, rushing to the place where we can retire and finally be happy.

We believe that your physical, mental, and emotional health compose the foundation to living a good life. If you make conscious decisions daily to take care of that, it will provide the foundation that leads you to a life of true happiness, one in which you enjoy both the journey and the destination.

START NOW

SMALL INVESTMENTS IN YOUR HEALTH EARLY ON PAY HUGE dividends later. It's just like saving for retirement. When you are young, it's really hard to do. Retirement seems so far off, and you really need the money now. It will be easier later on when you have more. Health is the same way. When you are young, it is just a given and so easily taken for granted. In both of these instances, it is so common to put it off till later, but so often later never comes. There is a Chinese proverb that states, "The best time to plant a tree was 20 years ago. The second-best time to plant a tree is today."

Although she worried, it wasn't too late for Sara, and it isn't too late for you either. Start today. The principles we are going to share over the next several chapters are filled with simple actions to help you start investing in your health NOW.

While these principles are simple, they aren't always easy. We may have the best of intentions, but those plans are often pushed aside, as we focus on keeping our head above the water, challenged with the day-to-day activities that seem so urgent (but not necessarily important) in the moment. One of Nate's favorite quotes is by Craig Groeschel, senior pastor of Life Church, best-selling author, and creator of *Craig Groeschel Leadership Podcast*. He says, "We don't drift to what is healthy. We drift to what is easy." We try so hard to stay on the right track but assuredly revert back to what is easy if we are not intentional. We are going to cover how to self-assess your current situation and what it takes to create a plan to help you become successful in creating the path that is right for you. So question two is, "Where do I want to go?"

ENJOY YOUR PATH

WE'VE COME TO THE CONCLUSION THAT THERE IS NO FINISH LINE to race to. It isn't better there than here. We don't want to wait until retirement to enjoy our life and live our dream. We want our cake and want to eat it too. And guess what? With planning and intentionality, we can have it all.

Have you ever looked to the future and envisioned what your life will be like, 10, 20, or even 30 years from now? Sorry, sitting on a beach drinking a margarita doesn't count. We glaze over the idea, thinking it's silly, but if we are in the driver's seat, why can't we control exactly where we want the bus to go? If you could map out your ideal day, not at retirement, but right now, what would it look like? Add in all the specifics, including the time you wake up, where you wake up, what you eat, and what you do for work. Yes, work is part of life, but for a fulfilling life we must find our passion and let it guide us. Work doesn't have to be a 9-to-5 where we check a box, literally clocking in and out every day. It can be something amazing! What sets your heart on fire and fills your cup? You want this to be a part of your ideal day. What else do you add in daily that balances it all out? What do your relationships look like? What type of people do enjoy being around? What do your afternoons and evenings look like? Do you have any hobbies? The more specific, the more intentional you can become in planning. Let's make a plan where you are kicking it into your nineties. What do you need to do daily to make this happen, and can you truly have it all?

The good news is that YES, we can have it all, but most of us won't get there without a good plan and a lot of intention supported with great habits. With intention and planning, we can have a long, meaningful lifespan AND an improved healthspan. The way we achieve true health is relatively simple. But remember, simple, my friend, isn't the same as easy. If it was easy, we would not have the health care crisis that we have in this country. What we now know is that small actions applied consistently compound over time to lead to huge results. It really is that simple.

Soon we'll dive into the five key factors of health, but first let's introduce you to Jake, Emma, Bob, and Carol, four friends who live similar lives but who have been doing things slightly differently over the years. As you'll see, those differences add up over time to create very divergent outcomes.

CHAPTER THREE
THE SECRET SAUCE

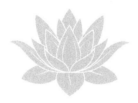

MEET BOB, CAROL, JAKE, AND EMMA

Bob and Carol met in college, fell in love, and got married after Bob finished graduate school. Bob works in corporate finance, and Carol is a third-grade teacher. In the early years of their relationship, life was filled with excitement and pleasure. They loved being active and were always up for adventures. They'd take weekend trips and do vigorous things like go hiking and kayaking. They felt so alive! During the regular workweek, Bob would hit the gym after work, and Carol would jog a few times per week.

A few years after being married, they had their first child, and two years later, the second came along. Life was turning out exactly as they had planned, and they had everything they wanted. They were living the American Dream and on the right path. It was so exciting in those early years, but as the kids grew older, the schedules became more and more hectic and priorities started to shift. The joy was still there, it just felt buried under responsibility most of the time. "Things are great, just busy," Carol would say when someone asked her how it was going. She loved being a mom. It came so naturally to her. Bob was a great dad too, but over the last 10 or so years, it seemed there was always a project or a promotion to be chasing at work that ate away at his physical and mental space. There just weren't enough hours in the day to find the time to prioritize healthy meals, good sleep, or exercise. They both had the best of intentions, but life just got in the way. Both Bob and Carol wished there was more time for their relationship and their personal health, but the kids were the priority. "We'll get back to taking care of 'us' someday," they both told themselves.

Their neighbors, Jake and Emma, followed a similar path. The two couples didn't meet each other until after college when they moved into houses across the street from each other. Carol brought some cookies over to welcome Jake and Emma to the neighborhood, and as they got acquainted, they couldn't believe how much the two families had in common. Jake and Emma had kids similar in age to Bob and Carol's daughters. In fact, the kids would be going to the same school in the fall. Jake and Emma were also busy professionals and feeling the strain from managing their work schedules along with the schedules of their three kids. Sometimes, first thing in the morning, when Bob was stumbling to the coffee pot half-awake, he'd see Jake outside in the total darkness. What in the heck was he doing?

When the two families met one weekend at the soccer field, Bob inquired, "Hey, I'm not a stalker, but I saw you outside early one morning this week. It was still dark outside. Not just dark, but pitch black. What in the heck were you doing?"

"Oh," Jake laughed. "I just got back from a run."

"Dude, it was still dark out. You're crazy," Bob scoffed.

Jake replied, "You have to pay yourself first, man. I find if I don't set time aside in the morning before most people get up, I get too busy with life demands, and I can't fit it in at all. You should join me sometime."

"Sure, maybe. One of these days when life slows down a bit," Bob replied.

LIFE WILL GET EASIER—SOMEDAY

CAN YOU RELATE TO THESE COUPLES? LIFE IS SO BUSY. AND without a lot of intention and considerable planning it is easy to let personal priorities slide. Often, we are so busy caring for everyone else that there is just no time to take care of ourselves. It feels kind of selfish, prioritizing our own needs. The world needs things from us, and we want to comply, fit in with the tribe, and do the acceptable things. By the time that is all done, we are too exhausted to do much for ourselves. We feel a tug, that we should be doing something proactive for ourselves, for our health, but we tell ourselves that someday we'll have time, which gives us some relief in the moment.

But here's the thing: when the kids are babies, we don't sleep, and we think it will be easier when they are toddlers. When they are toddlers, we are just surviving. My gosh, they never stop and the messes they make! And their energy—it's endless! It will DEFINITELY be easier when they start school. Then we're a slave to the school schedule and it's just plain busy—taxiing them everywhere—from school to soccer, to birthday parties and so much more. But good news, they'll be driving soon, then it will be easier. But then, when they are driving, we can't really sleep when they're out because we worry. So when exactly does it get easier?

The truth is, it doesn't get easier for a LONG time. And by the time it does, without prioritizing time for yourself and your marriage, it may be too late. But it doesn't have to be. With intention and planning, you can get off the default path of life and create an intentional life, living out your dreams. Those who have it didn't stumble upon it by accident. They regularly made small, consistent deposits in their "wellness" accounts and are reaping the benefits now. It's easy not to take this path. Most don't. Most won't.

It's really pretty simple, but don't confuse simple with easy. It's not the same. Not the same at all. It's especially hard because we don't see the benefits of our sacrifice for many years. We love instant results in today's society, right? Next-day shipping, information from the internet in seconds, DoorDash (when did we get too lazy to drive to get our fast food?), and movies on demand. Of course, we expect instant results when we start an exercise program or a diet—that's the way we've been conditioned. When we don't see the results quickly, we give up and think, "THIS isn't working. Maybe a different plan will work better." This is shiny object syndrome. The newest shiniest object (or exercise plan or fad diet) must surely be the better and the easier answer we are hoping for.

The truth is, even though you may not see it immediately—IT IS WORKING, you just need to give it more of the secret ingredient. The secret ingredient is good old-fashioned time.

So if you want to create a life of health so that you can thrive, not just survive, as the kids get older and move away, there are some simple (but not easy) things you can start to focus on today to get you there. Because the truth is, by the time life does get easier, without intention and planning, soccer games and birthday parties get replaced with doctors' appointments and tending to the wounds of poor health. The best years have passed you by.

True health is much more than acceptable blood pressure, OK cholesterol, and being up to date with your mammogram and colonoscopy. True health is having those test results at normal measures AND not just feeling OK but feeling great. When you are on a proactive path to optimal health, you have the confidence to know you have done your part to prevent chronic disease, and you are fulfilled because intuitively you know you're on your authentic path in life.

We are all on a journey. Bob and Carol are on the autopilot default path. They didn't consciously choose it, but they didn't consciously get off of this path either. Jake and Emma are purposefully choosing a different journey, a path of intention to get them to their optimal chosen purposeful destination.

FUNCTIONAL MEDICINE AND FUNCTIONAL FITNESS

FUNCTIONAL MEDICINE LOOKS TO FIND THE ROOT CAUSES OF THE symptoms patients present with. The goal in functional medicine is to fix the root cause rather than chasing symptoms and covering them up with medication. Instead of focusing on only what is wrong, functional medicine goes a step further and looks at why a body is responding the way it is. Our bodies are amazingly and intricately designed, and when things aren't functioning properly, there is a reason. Identifying the reason and fixing it are the keys to preventing and reversing chronic disease and optimizing health. This is accomplished by looking at tests beyond what traditionally trained doctors order and by looking for optimal, not just normal, results. Improving lifestyle plays a central role in functional medicine, and functional fitness is a large part of modifying lifestyle.

Functional fitness programs, like CrossFit, incorporate a lifestyle characterized by sound nutrition and functional movements, like focusing on exercises that help you with everyday activities such as getting up off the floor, carrying heavy objects, and putting something up on a shelf. Some people have the misconception that functional fitness programs like CrossFit are just for elite athletes, and that couldn't be farther from the truth. CrossFit movements are scalable to any ability level, and their foundational movements are ones we use in our everyday life. From a nutrition perspective they teach how to provide our body with the foods found naturally on earth and enough of them to provide energy to fuel our body for exercise but not body fat.

Both functional fitness and functional medicine focus on five factors of health:

1. Sleep
2. Diet
3. Exercise
4. Relationships
5. Mindset

Simple, but not easy, right? Truly focusing on these five factors every week leads to health and happiness and choices. You may decide you don't want to climb Mount Kilimanjaro when you are 70, but wouldn't it be nice to be able to if you decide you do want to?

NATE'S TAKE

AS WE GET OLDER, OUR LEVEL OF RESPONSIBILITY INCREASES, which usually means our ability to prioritize importance comes into play. Many adults—just like the couples previously mentioned—have the vision of living a long, healthy, abundant life, but what ends up happening? Ideally, they graduate from high school and are ready to tackle the "real world." For some, this may be heading to college, but for others it means going right into the workforce. No matter if it's in their late teens or mid-twenties, the individual steps into the tornado of adulthood. Some are more prepared than others. Some have had a much "easier path" than others. Either way, we could all agree, it's a challenging task. The mid-twenties rolls into the mid-thirties, and before we know it, we are in survival mode. Hours turn into days, days turn into years, and we blink our eyes and 20 years have passed by. It's as if we are living the same week a thousand times over and calling it a life.

Planning is something that sounds so simple but can be so challenging. "Stick to the plan" is another common catch phrase used in sports, military, and other social settings. The plan usually has the best interest of the team and individual in mind. A good plan has taken into account all the possible factors that could uproot your plan from being successful. So, while the five factors above look great and simple on paper, it ideally comes down to the planning of them into your day that determines how successful you are going to be.

Bob and Jake both can identify that some level of fitness is pretty important to their overall health. But what is the difference between the two men's daily routines? The difference all comes down to how they plan their day.

We must prepare to the level of a Navy Seal if we want to be truly successful. Navy Seals are one of the most well respected and decorated military groups of all time. Why are they so highly regarded, and why is their success rate so high? Why, when you hear that someone was a Navy Seal, does it instantly add a level of respect to that individual that is higher than if they were a former President of the United States? It is because they are the best of the best. They prioritize and execute. They make simple, yet detailed plans and execute them to the highest level. If the plan fails, they identify the shortcoming, take ownership of the failure, and put a new, better plan into action for the next time.

Libby, in functional medicine, and I, with CrossFit, have identified the five factors of health playing the ultimate role in a person's long-term health and wellness. If you can master these five areas, you will be truly living your best life.

Our goal in the pages to follow is to help you identify where you are at in each of the five factors, determine where you want to go in the future, and implement daily action steps to get you there. It's not a set-it-and-forget-it method. You'll continue to make adjustments fluidly as your life and goals change as the years pass.

STAY THE SAME OR DO SOMETHING?

THE AUTOPILOT PATH WON'T GET YOU WHERE YOU WANT TO GO, so to create a life on purpose, you have to steer your life in a specific direction.

Are you ready for an abundant life? A life where you not only feel great but have the confidence that you will have many choices presently and as you get older? A life where your retirement years won't be spent at doctors' appointments but instead with those you love the most and seeing the world? Being able to say YES to opportunities that come your way because you have health and vitality, and along with health and vitality come choices. Lots of choices.

Some people won't make changes in their health for themselves. Consider this—if we can't make the changes for ourselves, we can make it for our children. Living a life this way is modeling to our kids what true health looks like. The truth is, our kids learn so much more by what they see us do than what we tell them to do. Their little eyes are watching and listening and taking notes, so I think you should do it for yourself. But if you won't do it for yourself, do it for them. Some small sacrifices in the short term leads to great freedom in the long term. You are worth it. Your kids are worth it too.

Let's dive in and break down these five factors of health and get you on the path now. Let's start with a seemingly easy one—sleep!

CHAPTER FOUR

SLEEP—THE REAL BADGE OF HONOR

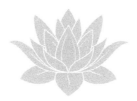

Sleep has gotten a bad rap, and it is often equated with laziness. "My lazy kid slept till noon." Or "I slept the day away and didn't accomplish anything." Contrast that with the badge of honor we apply to people who don't get a lot of sleep. "I only got three hours of sleep last night." Or "Sorry, I'm a little late, I pulled a double." We often admire those as scenarios of resilience and grit.

When I was in residency, I would work over 80 hours many weeks, frequently 36 hours in a row, and I too considered it a badge of honor. I was proud of the toughness associated with it. It was near the end of my residency in the early 2000s that residency work-hour restrictions were put into place following a highly publicized lawsuit where an 18-year-old patient died following the administration of a drug that interacted with one the patient was already taking. While it was concluded that the prescribing error was an innocent mistake, it sparked the development of a rule that is still in effect today: residents can work no more than 24 continuous hours and no more than 80 hours in a work week. This is still too much, but it is a step in the right direction.

Sleep is not just for lazy people. Sleep is very important, and getting this modifiable lifestyle factor right is essential to optimal health. Both the right quantity and good quality of sleep are paramount to feeling great. Sleep is the battery charger for our lives. Sleep is to your body as charging is to your phone.

Think of it like plugging your phone in before you go to bed at night. Ideally when you wake up, you pick up your phone and it is 100 percent charged. It is ready for a day of use. The body is no different. When your phone doesn't charge fully at night, problems occur. When you wake up and discover that has happened, you know you are going to have to modify your day to make the battery last. You do the same things with your body when you get poor sleep. What is your body's boost? Typically, it's coffee, energy drinks, or sugary foods throughout the day. These quick jump-start items are the same thing as plugging your phone into your car for a quick 10 to 15 minutes during a commute or carrying around your charger like it's your walking lifeline no matter where you go. This isn't a big deal if it happens rarely, but if getting poor sleep is the norm for you, the effects on your health can be devastating.

What if your phone was down to one percent, and instead of the seven hours it needs for a full charge, you could only charge it for two to three hours? What if your phone was almost out of battery power and instead of leaving it on the charger until it was fully charged, you unplugged it every 30 minutes and used it for 15 minutes before plugging it back into the charger? What could that do to the battery's lifespan? Even scarier, when you translate this example into our life and our sleep patterns, what's it doing to your lifespan and healthspan?

Great sleep is the foundation to building a great day. How often have you heard, when you have an important event on the horizon, "Make sure you get a good night's sleep"? Ideally, you should aim for this every evening of your life, not just when you have a big day to follow. When you get a good night's sleep, it starts the domino effect of positive action that leads to your daily health and wellness.

SLEEP—BOB AND JAKE

IT's MONDAY NIGHT, AND BOB AND JAKE MEET AGAIN, THIS TIME at the end of the driveway, taking the trash bins out for tomorrow's pickup day. Jake greets Bob with the ole "Hey, neighbor, how was your day?"

Bob, with an exhausted look and posture, responds, "Well, it was a Monday, that's for sure!"

Jake replies, "Oh, man, I'm guessing that means it wasn't very good?!"

Bob shrugs and explains, "Well, nothing catastrophic, just putting out fires all day at work, which leads to me playing catch-up on my computer later than I'd like tonight."

Jake responds with sincerity, "Yep, I have definitely been there before. Actually, Emma and I both have been there." Jake continued, "A couple of years ago, when Emma went back to work after having our youngest, we were burning it at both ends. With typical parental responsibilities, kids' practices, and work, we were walking around like a couple of zombies, not really loving life too much."

Nodding his head in agreement, Bob added, "No kidding. I feel like I am definitely in zombie land half the time."

They both shared a quick laugh.

Bob then added, "By the end of the week, I'm about as big of a walking zombie as it gets! It never seems to fail when I finally get caught up for the evening and turn on the game to have a beer, Carol *needs* me to do something."

Jake shook his head in agreement and replied, "Yeah, I understand what you're saying. Emma and I were definitely in that same boat a couple of years ago. When one evening, we looked at each other in exhaustion and anger after a long back-and-forth argument over something silly, I'm sure, and we both said, enough is enough, and something clicked for us."

Bob, standing there a bit intrigued, questioned, "Sooooo … what clicked? I'm up for any secrets of not being exhausted and arguing with Carol if you don't mind sharing. Did you hire a nanny?" He chuckled at his question.

Jake laughed, "No, but having another set of hands from time to time sure wouldn't hurt, huh?"

Bob replied, "Yeah, no kidding, or four sets of hands."

Jake then went on to explain, "No, but in all seriousness, Emma I looked at each other after that argument a few years back, and said to each other, 'Why are we even arguing and mad at each other again? This makes no sense.' We realized that at the end of the day, our relationship with each other and the kids was the most important thing. Working into the evenings was causing most of the issues. We decided to write down some non-negotiables together that would hopefully help eliminate our struggles in the evenings with one another."

Bob, who seemed really interested now, asked, "What do you mean by 'non-negotiables'?"

Jake went on, "Well, they are just a few simple rules that we follow every night as a family, that help eliminate the snapback arguments with one another. We both came to the understanding that the kids and each other come first in our lives. Now we have to start setting boundaries when work can get in the way of that."

Bob responded sarcastically, "Oh, I get ya, nothing like adding some more rules to your marriage."

Jake laughed and said, "Yeah, it may seem like that, but it's actually pretty simple. We agreed to no devices or work after 7:30 p.m., so we can spend time with the kids winding down for the evening, and lights out at 9:30 to make sure we are well rested up for the following day."

Bob questioned, "So you never do anything work-related after 7:30? That would be a dream!"

Jake explained, "It was challenging for sure at first, but once you both establish it as a non-negotiable and realize it helps you be the parents and spouse you want to be, it's not as challenging. Sure, every once in a while something might come up that may need my attention for a few minutes, but that has only happened once or twice over the last couple of years. As I see it, people need to rest and recharge, and the nighttime is when that happens … Well, I'd love to hang out and chat, but that alarm rings awfully early in the morning, so I better head in, so I can get my seven hours!" Jake then added, "If you ever want to join me in the morning for a run, Bob, it's an open invite. I'd love to have a partner."

Bob responded, "Yeah, maybe someday. I think I better start with the house rule list with Carol first. She's gonna love this one."

Bob walked back towards the house with mixed emotions. Jake's insight had him asking himself a number of questions. "Do I really need any more rules in my life? Heck, all I do is follow rules, rules at work, rules in marriage, rules in parenting, rules as an adult. Pretty sure the last thing I need is a list of nightly rules at home as well. But then again if it means turning off my computer and not waking up feeling like a zombie … heck, might be worth a try."

With all of life's demands, it isn't easy to prioritize sleep. However, it is important and there are devastating consequences if you routinely sleep less than six to seven hours per night. Let's dive in and see the benefits of good sleep, the downsides of poor sleep, and what common things interfere with our ability to get a good night's sleep.

DR. LIBBY'S TOP 10 SLEEP TIPS

Tip 1—Make it a priority to get a good night's sleep because it helps your immune system.

Poor sleep suppresses the immune system. Actually, poor sleep doesn't just suppress your immune system, it can actually demolish your immune system. Translation: you get sick more easily and have a harder time getting over it.

Tip 2— Make it a priority to get a good night's sleep in order to have better appetite control.

Poor sleep makes you hungry. Poor sleep elevates blood sugar and increases hunger—both are problematic if you have weight to lose or struggle with insulin resistance (like patients with type 2 diabetes, prediabetes, or polycystic ovarian syndrome).

Tip 3— Make it a priority to get a good night's sleep to help decrease your risk of chronic disease.

Poor sleep leads to chronic disease. Lack of sleep increases the risk of depression, anxiety, Alzheimer's disease, heart disease, stroke, congestive heart failure, and even doubles your risk of cancer.

We don't just sleep to avoid the above-mentioned negative consequences. There are also many pro-health effects of a good night's sleep.

Tip 4— Make it a priority to get a good night's sleep to support your emotional wellbeing.

A good night's sleep resets our emotional circuits—essential for a happy and productive next day. Now it makes sense why teens need so much sleep!

Tip 5— Make it a priority to get a good night's sleep to support the health of your gut.

Sleep maintains our microbiome—this is the "good bacteria" that live in our gut that provide many positive health benefits. About one trillion bacteria live in the gut. Some of these bacteria are beneficial and do things like aid in digestion, support the immune system, regulate blood sugar, and produce neurotransmitters regulating brain health. "Bad bacteria" can lead to negative health consequences like weight gain, heart disease, and gastrointestinal problems such as irritable bowel syndrome or inflammatory bowel disease. The good bacteria help to push out the bad bacteria, so anything we can do to support our good gut bacteria is good for our overall health. A good night's sleep is good for our good gut bacteria.

Tip 6—Maintain a consistent sleep schedule in order to support your circadian rhythm and enhance your health.

Maintaining a circadian rhythm is health-enhancing. We all have a 24-hour internal clock. This is our circadian rhythm, and it's so important to optimal health to have a proper circadian rhythm. It is so important, in fact, that elite CrossFit coach, author, and podcaster Ben Bergeron suggests that if we work a second or third shift job, it is so detrimental to our health that we should quit and find a new job. Wow! That's extreme, but I see his point. Our body was designed to be awake and alert in the daylight hours and resting in the dark hours. Deviating from this leads to negative health consequences. Shift work has negative consequences, including an increased risk for high blood pressure, elevated blood sugar, elevated cholesterol, and an increased risk of obesity, heart disease, and stroke. Shift work leads to a decreased lifespan! If you have a job that prevents you from honoring your natural circadian rhythm and quitting isn't an option, there are some things you can do to mitigate the negative effects.

First of all, it's important to maintain sleep consistency, essentially going to bed at the same time and waking up at the same time, even on your days off. Your body really wants to be in a rhythm. Also make your room as dark as possible for sleep by using black-out curtains or an eye mask. Exposing yourself to bright light upon awakening will also help to establish this rhythm by signaling your brain that it is now time to be awake and alert. Despite these modifications, shift work remains a challenge that the body wasn't designed to handle. Do the best you can do.

Tip 7—Limit or avoid caffeine, especially after 2 p.m.

Caffeine can have profound effects on your ability to get a good night's sleep. In addition to the 24-hour internal clock, there is another system that determines whether you are asleep or awake—completely independent of the 24-hour internal clock. It's called sleep pressure. After you wake up in the morning, a chemical called adenosine begins to accumulate in your brain. The more it accumulates, the sleepier you become. Caffeine displaces adenosine from the receptors in the brain—leading to increased alertness. However, even while the caffeine is on board, adenosine still accumulates, so when the caffeine wears off, the adenosine floods the receptors, often resulting in an immense need to sleep. Also, the half-life of caffeine is five to six hours. So if you drink a cup of coffee at 3 p.m., at 9 p.m., half of the caffeine is gone, but half of it is still in your system. This can have big effects on your ability to get a good night's sleep.

Tip 8—Don't freak out if you don't sleep through the night.

Understand that no one sleeps through the night. We sleep in 90-minute sleep intervals. It often seems like we sleep through the night because there is just a brief awakening between these intervals. Generally, you have to be awake for one to two minutes to remember it the next day. Early on in the night, these 90-minute cycles consist mostly of non-rapid eye movement (NREM) sleep. NREM sleep is the deep, restorative sleep. In the second half of your sleep hours, rapid eye movement (REM) sleep predominates. This type of sleep is commonly referred to as dream sleep. During REM sleep, memory and learning are strengthened.

Tip 9—Don't go to bed too late or get up too early.

There are negative effects of going to bed too late and other negative effects of getting up too early, both of which provide equal but different devastating consequences. If you go to bed late, you lose out on a large percentage of the deep restorative (NREM) sleep. Also, the brain has its own waste management system, called the glymphatic system, where waste products that accumulate from energy breakdown get flushed out at night during sleep. This brain cleanup happens during NREM sleep, and you miss out on this important function by staying up too late. Conversely, if you get up too early, you lose out on a large proportion of REM sleep—making memory and learning more challenging. It's so important to have enough of both types of sleep to achieve optimal health and performance.

Tip 10—Limit or avoid drinking alcohol, especially at night.

Alcohol significantly disrupts natural sleep. Alcohol is a sedative, like sleeping pills, so it sedates you out of wakefulness but does not induce natural sleep. So even though you feel sedated, you aren't actually sleeping better. Sleep is more fragmented (more frequent awakenings) with alcohol on board. Also, alcohol is a powerful suppressor of REM sleep and, therefore, has negative effects on memory and learning.

As you can see, there are amazing benefits to getting a great night's sleep and destructive consequences to consistently poor sleep. A lot of really important cleanup is happening while we sleep, so it definitely isn't just for lazy people and underachievers. Some of our favorite beverages during the afternoon (coffee) and evening (alcohol) can have damaging effects on our sleep quality. Remember, there are two important factors to consider when evaluating your overall sleep—the quantity of sleep you are getting (the number of hours) and the quality of the sleep you are getting.

NATE'S TAKE: DESIGNING YOUR PLAN

PLANNING IS AN IMPORTANT PIECE OF THE PUZZLE, IF NOT THE most important piece of the puzzle. It was Ben Franklin who coined the phrase, "Failure to plan is planning to fail." A more present-day author of the New York Times bestseller *Atomic Habits,* James Clear states, "People do not rise to the level of their goals but fail to the level of their systems." If planning was so important in success in the 1700s and still is today, we must ask ourselves, "How can I plan well when it comes to sleep?"

What does the system look like that ensures that we are meeting our individual goals? In regard to sleep and the other factors of health and wellness that follow, every individual will have their own goal and definition of success. As time progresses and our habits improve and life begins to change, we will change our plan much like the peewee football player and NFL athlete have altered their pre-game rituals over the years. When it comes to the five factors, we have to identify our individual goals and needs to meet where we are currently at. Once we have done a quick self-assessment, we can then design a plan that meets us where we are at as individuals.

There are four basic steps that we are going to follow when it comes to the five areas of health. The key factor to remember is that these are not set-it-and-forget-it type of steps. Just as a healthy business does not wait until the fourth quarter to find out if they have won or lost for the year, we should not wait until the end of the month or even the end of the year to see where we fell short. This will be a recurring process where we can evaluate ourselves, on a scale from one to four and four to one. We need to look at this weekly and see where adjustments need to be made. Was it a poor plan, poor execution, or maybe a combination of both?

YOUR SLEEP PLANNING

1. Self-assessment—Where am I currently at?
2. Create a plan—Where am I trying to go?
3. Implementation of plan—Put plan in motion, daily discipline.
4. Tracking—Is my plan working?

Goal: For an adult, age 18 and above, the goal is seven to nine hours of sleep nightly.

Sleep is probably the easiest of the factors to plan across all ages, genders, and health and wellness levels because it is pretty standard in comparison to diet, exercise, relationships, and mindset work. For sleep there can nearly be a one-size-fits-all approach.

There are many ways to calculate and dissect your level of sleep. Using technology—like an Apple watch, **WHOOP**, Fitbit, or any other digital health tracker—can be an extremely effective way to track the amount and quality of your sleep. There are also less expensive techniques that you can use to track the metrics related to sleep. Think of it as simply as if you are in bed for eight hours, head to a pillow, then your body is probably getting the seven hours that is needed. There are a million other scenarios, but this is a general guideline and starting point. Let's not get caught in majoring in the minors. To start, it's pretty simple. Ask yourself, were you in bed for eight hours? Did you sleep fairly soundly? If you did, then without overcomplicating things, you can safely assume you got at least seven hours of sleep.

Sounds pretty simple, but in order to do it effectively, how do we plan it so we don't fail? Let's look at our couples and see what their plans look like.

Bob Goal: Bob needs seven hours of sleep, eight hours with his head on a pillow.

Bob's Evening

Bob gets home around 7 p.m. from the day's activities that are commonly encountered in life and parenthood. As soon as he walks through the door, Bob heads straight to his office.

Bob checks his email and takes care of some loose ends from work, so they are not on his plate first thing the next morning. He makes a vow to be off of his computer by 8 p.m. even though he still has some work things he would love to take care of. He signs off at 8 p.m. and grabs a plate of dinner that Carol has ordered in. The family spreads out throughout the house while eating dinner. Carol sits with the youngest to minimize the disaster that can come with a toddler during dinner time. Their oldest is watching her favorite YouTube program while eating with her plate on the living room floor while Bob sits in front of the TV with some of his favorite pizza and a beer to catch the beginning of the Thursday night football game. The kids finish up their dinner, and Carol takes the lead getting the kids wound down for the evening and ready for bed. Both kiddos give their dad a kiss goodnight before they head off to bed by 9 p.m.

Bob stays up to watch the first half of the game while thumbing through his phone until 10:15 p.m. when he calls it for the night. Bob makes quick work of the kids' half-finished dinner plates, then does a speedy cleanup of the kitchen, so Carol doesn't have to in the morning. Bob completes the pre-bedtime routine and joins Carol in bed where he does some social media scrolling before hitting the lights and calling it a night a little before 11 p.m.

"This is exactly what Jake was talking about," Bob thinks to himself. "My head on a pillow from 11 p.m. to a 7 a.m. alarm, that will give me eight hours in bed which ensures the seven hours of sleep. I crushed it!" Bob thinks to himself.

Goal: Jake needs seven hours of sleep—eight hours with his head on a pillow.

Across the street, Jake and Emma get home around the same time from their kids' soccer practice as their neighbors do. Within 15 to 20 minutes of walking in the door, dinner is served up from a crockpot meal on the table by 7:30 p.m. Even with a few small adjustments for the girls' special interests in food, the family finishes up around 8:15 with dinner. As a family, they sit down together and share conversations and time together. They discuss their day's wins and losses from school, work, and practices.

Jake and Emma make quick work of cleaning up the kitchen together and have the kids bathed and ready for bed by 8:45. It's a divide-and-conquer kind of night. Jake lies in bed with the older two to read a chapter of their favorite book while Emma lies in bed with the youngest for some quick cuddles to help her fall asleep. By 9 p.m. the kids are well on their way to sleep and Jake and Emma get ready for bed. Before they hit the lights, they have a quick chat about plans for tomorrow to confirm responsibilities on who is taking who where, just to make sure there are no hiccups in the morning.

What's the Difference?

First of all, both families are doing a great job. The goal here is evaluating where you are and making small improvements to move closer to a better lifestyle, better health, and a better life. It's essential to ensure you are taking more steps forward than backward when it comes to health. To someone that is only getting four to five hours of sleep, Bob's "plan" is a pretty good one, compared to having no plan at all. If we were starting with someone who is not even close to getting the seven actual hours, then Bob's plan is a great starting point. But if we want to live the longest, healthiest life possible, then we should plan like we are in the big leagues.

Think of it again as a comparison to football. In peewee football there are two to three coaches that help run the team together, usually volunteers. They make a game plan at practice, go over some of the small stuff, like drills, plays to run on offense based on personnel, and some other basic defensive strategies. However, as the children progress in age and skill, the coaching level increases from the volunteer to eventually a career professional. When the children progress from peewee, junior high, high school, college, and the highest level of professional, the plan gets more and more dialed-in each step of the way. Every position has its own set of paid professional coaches. The organization typically even has its own team of professionals that focus on strength, nutrition, sleep, and psychological wellness. Some would argue that these areas have no direct skill connection with the sport, so why have paid staff to "pamper" the players in these areas? As the professionals know, the difference between making it to the Super Bowl and having a losing record is in the details! So the better we want to be, the longer we want to live, then the better our plan must be.

Some people might want to live their lives with fewer rules and planning. Some want to have drinks during the week, get the five to seven hours of sub-par sleep, and party it up every weekend. Individuals that fall into that category are probably good with Bob's sleep plan. That is 100 percent fine.

Bob's decisions above will probably get him to the average lifespan in the United States. However, his lifespan may exceed his healthspan. Simply put, he may be alive longer than he'll be healthy and independent. In this case, there are probably years of life where he's going to need assistance to complete daily tasks in order to survive. Some of those years might be spent in assisted living or by depending on family or friends for his activities of daily living.

Bob's plan is a C at best. Overindulging in food before bed, drinking alcohol, letting the mind wander on work tasks not completed, and overstimulating the mind with TV all lead to poorer sleep. Drinking 20 to 30 ounces of anything before bed means one to two bathroom trips in the middle of the night, especially as you age. All of these things do not seem like much by themselves, but when you start combining them, they create a poor sleep cocktail that is hard to fight. The majority of Americans have fallen into a similar situation.

RATE YOURSELF AND CREATE A SLEEP PLAN

IF YOU WANT TO CONTINUE TO GROW AS AN INDIVIDUAL AND improve in all areas of life, then you need to create healthy sleep habits now that will keep you on the path of intention in your journey for optimal health and your best life.

There is no one-size-fits-all recipe for the perfect diet, sleep, exercise, relationships, and mindset strategies. It must be one that is created for you that matches your goals and lifestyle.

Just like compound interest, the more you invest in sleep and the other factors of health in your earlier years by making healthy deposits like Jake and Emma, the more opportunities you will have when you get into later years. It seems counterintuitive, but the more rigid you are with rules and caring for yourself in the present, the more freedom and choices you actually create for yourself in the future.

While creating healthy habits is the key to success for your health and wellness bank account, it is best to keep in mind realistic expectations for each of those areas. You want to set goals that are achievable but will still be somewhat challenging. These daily action steps will be the foundation that you will build and grow upon as you get better at planning and becoming more disciplined. The plan we recommend for all of the five factors is going to be a series of small daily decisions in each area that you are going to build over time. These small deposits will compound over time creating a happier, healthier you.

Remember, just because these suggestions are simple, that doesn't mean they are easy. They can take some time to work. Stick with it. The road less traveled is worth it. You can let your primitive brain that is wired for survival take control and get the results that most people do OR you can do something more purposeful. You can look to the evolved portion of your brain, plan a life on purpose, and become the hero of your own story. First assess where you are currently, and then we'll guide you to create a plan to get where you want to be.

SLEEP—RATE YOURSELF

Rate yourself from 1   2   3   4   5   6   7   8   9   10

(With 1 being two to three hours of interrupted sleep and 10 being ten hours of uninterrupted sleep.)

My Bedtime Routine:
Before I go to bed, I typically _____,
_____, _____.

Level 1—Rating 1–3

If you are at the bottom on the far left of the "Sleep—Rate Yourself" number line, let's start with a few basic items to see if we can't get your score of 1 to 3 up to a 4 to 5. The good news is there are some small changes that you can make that should make a big difference in a relatively small window of time. At the end of the chapter, there is a chart that has the basic idea of deposits and withdrawals when it comes to your health savings account. The more deposits you have, the more you are "investing" in your health just like making deposits into a retirement account.

Three great practices to start with include the following:
- Having a technology cut-off time
- Eliminating alcohol
- Creating a bedtime routine

Just like your bank account, the goal is to have more deposits than withdrawals. Start with an inventory of where you are currently. Are you overdrawn on your sleep account to start? Once you have established a baseline, keep track of these daily. Your brain focuses on what you track, and tracking more likely leads to success!

Level 2—Rating 4–6

If you are in the 4 to 6 range, you can just build on what was done in the last step. If you successfully implemented three steps, can you add two to three more into that routine? Look at the list of deposits and withdrawals when it comes to sleep. Try adding a few more deposits or removing a few more withdrawals. The list isn't inclusive, so feel free to add something that isn't on that list if it seems applicable to you and your situation. Identify where the struggles are. Is the problem physically getting into bed for enough hours? Or are you devoting enough time to sleep, but the sleep is interrupted? If the issue is that you are not in bed long enough, that is fairly simple. You just have to set boundaries to what you are doing in the evenings to make sure that your sacred recharge time is prioritized. It is a big deal and you are worth it.

Think of it like putting an event in your calendar for a meeting that you cannot cancel. It is honorable to show up for the event you have committed to, and I bet you do just that. But what about when the commitment is to yourself, like going to bed at a certain time? Do you honor your commitments to yourself too, just like you honor your commitments to others? This is a bigger struggle for most of us. If the issue is quality of sleep, then we might have to do more investigation. Are you getting up to go to the bathroom? If so, cut out liquids earlier. Is it a full stomach that is causing you to toss and turn? If so, choose meals wisely, considering both the quantity and quality of the food. Also ensure adequate time to digest the food before bed. Sometimes something as easy as adding in a little 15- to 20-minute walk right after eating can be enough to help kick start digestion.

Maybe you, like many people, fall asleep easily but then wake up long before the alarm goes off and can't turn your mind off. The tasks that lie ahead of you are weighing you down. How about journaling those things down before bed or even when you are stuck awake. This helps to reset and make sure they are not forgotten. Our brains are actually not designed to store information but rather to process it, so jotting the things down that you are worried you may forget is a big relief for your brain and will likely help you fall back to sleep.

Level 3—Rating 7–10

This is a great number, and you should be happy with this. It means six to seven nights a week you are getting eight hours in bed, which ensures the seven hours of solid sleep. Are there ways you could get better? Absolutely! If you are already at this level, you may consider a sleep monitoring device like an Apple watch, Whoop, Fitbit, Polar Vantage, Biostrap EVO, or similar product. These will not only tell you the number of hours you sleep, but they will also rate your quality of sleep. This adds valuable information beyond the simple calculation of the number of hours your head is on the pillow.

Beware, sometimes adding an electronic monitoring system will consume you and cause negative effects. When it comes to fitness or sleep, sometimes you can become addicted to the results or what the watch is saying that you did or did not do. You may become more consumed with the data these devices provide than the benefits of the exercise or sleep itself. Just remember, waking up alert and refreshed is a better indicator of the quality of your sleep than any watch will ever be able to tell you. You are the expert on you. If the results on the device conflict with the results you are personally seeing, go with YOU every time.

Below are great indicators that can help you gauge sleep quality without fancy gadgets.

What is your quality? If you hit all these indicators, then you are probably doing just fine.

- ☯ You fall asleep soon after getting into bed, within 30 minutes or less.
- ☯ You typically sleep straight through the night, waking up no more than once per night.
- ☯ You're able to sleep the recommended number of hours for your age group (7–9 hours for all adults).
- ☯ If you do wake up, you fall back asleep within 20 minutes.
- ☯ You feel rested, restored, and energized upon waking up in the morning.

If you are hitting all these markers, then you are exactly where you need to be. It is best to note that you can use your device to measure the time in bed and total hours slept, but just because it doesn't give you a good grade on your sleep markers—like HRV, sleep cycles, regeneration, and other markers—it does not mean you are not getting good sleep. Just like anything else, technology does malfunction, and not all sleep trackers are created equal. True sleep tests are done by measuring your brain waves, the oxygen level in your blood, heart rate, and breathing, as well as eye and leg movements. All of these markers are beyond what a watch will do for you.

Are you ready to start tracking? For amazing health, not every step needs to be forward, but you do need to have more steps forward than backwards. We pay attention to what we track. Please go to www.thepathofinention.com to download a free companion tracker guide to start tracking your sleep and the other modifiable lifestyle factors today.

Managing your sleep is prioritizing your health and moves you from the autopilot default path to the path of intention for improved health. You've got this!

Daily Sleep Deposits (+)	Daily Sleep Withdrawals (–)
Exercising daily for 45–60 minutes.	Exercising late in the evening (less than two hours before bedtime)
Turning off devices one hour before bed	Eating a late meal (less than two hours before bedtime)
Establishing a pre-sleep routine—three things you automatically do to signal your brain it's time for sleep (e.g., wash face, brush teeth, get morning coffee ready)	Going to bed angry at someone
Reading before bed	Bedtime varying by more than 1 hour from night to night
Drinking calming tea at night	Drinking alcohol
Using a white noise machine	Checking social media or email first thing the next morning
Exposing yourself to natural (or 10,000 lux) light within 30 minutes of waking for the day	Using the snooze button
Cutting off your caffeine intake by 2 p.m.	Watching TV in the bedroom before bed
Doing a next-morning checklist before bedtime (a list of things to do the next day, so you aren't worrying about forgetting something)	Napping excessively during the day (greater than 45 minutes)
Engaging in intimacy with partner	Playing on phone before bed
Having a hot bath prior to bed	Watching news 30 minutes before bed

Disclaimer: trying something once or twice, then claiming it doesn't work doesn't count. It has to be an honest effort over an extended period of time.

SLEEP ACTION STEPS

Current Sleep Rating is a _____ of 10

Three action steps for improvement are:

1._____

2._____

3._____

What is one small change you can make today in regards to your sleep? Consistency carves canyons, and every step forward is a step to better health. The little things matter!

Are you ready to tackle what we consider to be the most complicated of the five factors—diet? Let's go there next.

CHAPTER FIVE

DIET—YOU CAN'T OUTWORK A
BAD ONE

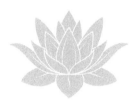

No One-Size-Fits-All

Are you ready for the bad news? I'm just going to give it to you—right out of the gate. There is no one diet to follow, no one-size-fits-all that you can easily implement today and be on the correct path forward forever. Each body is unique and complicated. When thinking about dieting, think about FOREVER, instead of FAST. Remember, the tortoise wins the race, not the hare.

Have you ever been on a diet where you quickly lost weight only to gain it back over the next several months? This yo-yo dieting wreaks havoc on your metabolism. You should be more interested in changes in your diet that are sustainable for the long term in your quest for optimal health. When you focus on the metric of health, instead of weight loss, the weight loss follows in a slower, but more sustainable fashion. You don't lose weight and get healthy. It's the other way around. You get healthy, and the weight loss then follows, slowly but surely.

Emma and Carol

Emma goes to the grocery store every weekend after she and Jake chat about what their week will look like and they decide what they'd like to eat. They check the pantry, fridge, and freezer to see what they already have and make a list of what they will need. On Sunday afternoons they prepare as much as they can ahead of time. They chop veggies, clean the fruit, and prepare the protein. It's all ready to go. Emma no longer buys the things she used to crave. It wasn't easy in the beginning, but now that she's detoxed her body from sugar, she rarely thinks about it anymore. The weekends are a little different for Jake, Emma, and the kids. They usually go out on Friday or Saturday night or both. They have what they want, but never really overindulge. Sometimes pizza sounds great, and they'll have just that. They feel good about loosening the reins a little on the weekends because they've done so well during the week.

Carol goes to the grocery store several times each week. She'd love to plan meals, but they are just so darn busy with the kids' activities. By the time she gets home from work, she's tired, and nothing really sounds good. They rush the kids to practice—Bob going in one direction and Carol in the other. Sometimes Bob picks up fast food for everyone on his way home. Other nights, they have cereal or something quick they can heat up in the microwave. Carol feels guilty and wishes she had a better grasp on diet for herself and her family. She expresses her concern to Bob one night prior to bed.

He reassures her that they'll do better once life slows down a little bit. There just isn't time to eat healthy with all they have on their plate right now. Surely it will be easier in the future, they hope.

Tonight, they have a sitter and are going out to dinner with Jake and Emma. The last time they went out, about a month ago, Bob teased Jake and said, "What are you going to have, Jake? The brussels sprout and kale salad with a side of lemon water?" Jake laughed and said he hadn't decided yet. Bob was shocked when Jake ordered a burger, sweet potato fries, and a beer. Emma ordered something similar. Bob found himself feeling a little envious of Jake—it didn't seem fair that he could eat that type of food and still maintain his weight and health. That was such a struggle for Bob. Some people have all the luck!

YOU ARE WHAT YOU EAT

YOU ARE WHAT YOU EAT. YOUR BODY IS CONSTANTLY RECYCLING old cells and creating new ones. "What materials is my body using to create these new cells?" you may ask. The building blocks come from the food you choose to feed it, so these new cells that your body is creating can be built with Oreos and potato chips OR with healthy fats, lean protein, and a wide array of nutrients from a rainbow of fruits and veggies. The difference between these two paths of vastly different building materials is huge, in your overall health and the way you feel.

We live in a world today where, without a lot of intention and planning, it's so easy to be "overfed and undernourished." In fact, in 2014, Netflix chronicled the toll that this global epidemic of the modern lifestyle is taking on our overall health in a documentary with this same title. A calorie isn't a calorie. Yes, calories will determine your overall weight to a certain extent, but what the calories are made of is critically important.

Your body is a very complex system that needs many essential vitamins, minerals, and nutrients to function at their best. Diet is complicated. The truth is, for optimal health you have to not only eat the right food, but you also have to eat the right amount of food for your activity level, digest it properly, and have a healthy gut to absorb the nutrients from those high-quality foods. And if that isn't enough to worry about, you also have to consider the nutritional content of the foods being produced these days. The soil that many of these foods are grown in is often depleted of essential nutrients. Additionally, due to the chemicals sprayed on crops, the resulting grains, fruits, and vegetables have toxins on them, which can be damaging to the liver and hence your health.

Let's not get hung up on the small details. There are some key principles with diet that if you choose to live by, will absolutely set you up for success. Focus on these big key concepts, and you'll be well on your way to having this modifiable lifestyle factor in the bag.

Dr. Libby's Top 10 Tips for Eating Healthy

Tip 1—Eat real food.

Real food is the stuff found on the perimeter of the grocery store. This is the stuff that goes bad in your fridge or pantry if you don't eat it quickly. If it can live in your pantry for months or even years, there are preservatives in it, allowing it to do so. Those preservatives aren't good for you. These foods are often highly processed, and their nutritional value has been stripped. Your body wasn't designed to process ingredients that you can't even pronounce.

Tip 2—Veggies, veggies, and more veggies.

The more veggies you eat, the better. Each vegetable has essential nutrients, and each one has different essential nutrients. A wide variety helps keep all of your health pathways working optimally. You are what you eat! What about fruits? Well, fruits are good too. Eating a rainbow of colors is great for your health. Just remember, fruits have natural sugar in them—so they are a treat, not something to be consumed in large quantities daily. Think of fruit as a dessert, something to be enjoyed in small quantities at the end of the meal.

Tip 3—Eat lots of fiber.

There is a lot you can track with your diet. Fiber is one of the most important. Fiber is the part of plant-based foods that passes through your digestive system without breaking down or being digested. Aim to get 25 to 50 grams of fiber each and every day. Most Americans are FAR under this goal, by the way. I think this is the most important thing to track. There are two types of fiber—insoluble and soluble fiber. Insoluble fiber attracts water into the stool, making it easier to pass with less strain. Insoluble fiber also increases the gut transit rate, which is the time it takes for food to move from the mouth all the way through the intestines, so it's good for helping with constipation. The other type of fiber, soluble fiber, actually creates a gel that may improve digestion. This gel can patch leaky areas in the gut lining. Also, soluble fiber breaks down into products called short-chained fatty acids, which are fuel for the microbiome (our good gut bacteria). In addition to normalizing bowel movements, fiber also lowers cholesterol, helps control blood sugar, aids in achieving a healthy weight, and helps you live longer by decreasing the risk of cardiovascular disease and all cancers. The average American eats about 10 to 15 grams of fiber per day, so there is lots of room for improvement here.

Tip 4—Drink lots of water.

Water is the single most important nutrient. Our cells are 70 percent water. That's a lot! Water constitutes 90% of our blood, which is how oxygen is delivered from the lungs to the rest of our body. Water also flushes body waste, lubricates the joints, helps maintain blood pressure, and aids in digestion. According to the USDA, the average American consumes 3.9 cups of water per day or 31.2 ounces. Most people need at least double that amount of water. Too much water can lead to imbalances in your electrolytes, so don't go crazy here. Hyponatremia (which is the fancy doctor term for low sodium) can be life-threatening. A good rule of thumb is to take your body weight in pounds and divide it by two and aim for that many ounces of water per day.

Tip 5—Stop buying low fat.

This is hard to get used to. We are so conditioned to worry about calories, and fat does have the most calories per gram. However, when the fat is missing, remember something else is taking its place. Something else is present to keep the food tasting good and keep consumers buying it and eating it. Usually that something else is sugar or an equally unhealthy derivative of sugar. Be careful. The food labels can be tricky because sugar can be called more than 50 different things. Low fat isn't the easy solution we thought it was going to be when this craze became popular in the 1980s and 1990s. Sugar is to blame for disease—not fat—and the low-fat phenomenon has led to an epidemic of diabetes and obesity.

Fat is a major source of energy. It helps absorb some vitamins and minerals. It is needed to build cell membranes and form sheaths around nerves.

Not all fat is the same, though, so here's the scoop. Think of fats as "bad," "in-between," and "good." Bad fat is trans-fat. It was banned in the US in 2018. It increases inflammation, which is a huge driver for chronic disease. Be careful because often a food label will say, "No trans-fat." If there is less than 0.5 grams per serving in a food, it can be advertised as "No trans-fat." To be safe, avoid these foods: shortening, microwave popcorn, margarine, vegetable oils, fried fast foods, bakery products, and non-dairy coffee creamers. Look for the words, "partially hydrogenated oil," on the label, and if it's there, this is a food you should avoid.

"In-between" fat is saturated fat. It is found in red meat, whole milk, cheese, and coconut oil. This is OK to eat in moderation.

Good fat consists of both mono- and polyunsaturated fats. Monounsaturated fats are found in olive oil, avocado, and nuts. Polyunsaturated fats are found in fatty fish, flax seeds, and walnuts. Polyunsaturated fats are essential, meaning the body needs them to function properly but cannot make them on its own, so you need to get them from your diet. Eating polyunsaturated fats in place of saturated fats or highly refined carbs decreases LDL (bad cholesterol) and triglycerides and improves the overall cholesterol profile.

Tip 6—FAST.

You do this already. You fast from the last calorie you put in your mouth before you go to bed until you take in the first calorie in the morning after waking. Actually, the word "breakfast" means "breaking the fast." I'm sure you've heard breakfast is the most important meal of the day, right? Well, it is believed that this slogan was created in the 1900s by John Harvey Kellogg, and his motive was selling breakfast cereals. So, yes, it is the most important meal of the day if your goal is selling breakfast cereal!

While you fast, your gut is resting, and this is helpful for recycling old damaged cells, reducing inflammation, enhancing detoxification, and improving brain health. These benefits can happen with just 12 hours of fasting. For example, you would be fasting for 12 hours if you ate your last meal at 7 p.m. and you don't eat again until 7 a.m. Totally doable.

When you fast, your insulin level gets low. A low insulin level triggers the body to burn fat for fuel. A high insulin level, on the other hand, triggers fat storage. Having a low insulin level is both health-promoting and weight-loss-promoting.

There are many variations of intermittent fasting, each with different eating and fasting windows, but the basic premise is the same. There is an eating window during which you consume your food and a fasting window in each variation. Fasting is natural, and our ancestors did it unintentionally due to limited access to food. Think about this. Our body fat is stored fuel for later use. The problem is, we don't get around to using it if we are always eating. Fasting is an opportunity to burn that stored fuel.

Fasting isn't a diet. It doesn't change WHAT you eat, but instead changes WHEN you eat. It's a pattern of eating that's beneficial to your health. And it's free! No one markets intermittent fasting because there is nothing to sell, which makes the benefits all the more trustworthy.

Tip 7—Limit sugar and flour.

With white flour, the beneficial part of the whole grain has been removed. The fine powder that is created by the grinding of the grain into flour spikes the blood sugar, which spikes the insulin. Really, when it comes to health, it's best to avoid the four white powders: sugar, flour, salt, and cocaine. Yes, you read that correctly, I lumped in sugar with cocaine. Many people are sugar addicts. For addicts, a little bit is too much, and a lot is never enough. If this is you—you are best to AVOID sugar, not just limit it. We would never tell a cocaine addict that it's OK to have a little bit of cocaine, just on the weekends, as long as they get back on track on Monday.

Tip 8—Buy organic. It's worth the extra money.

Organic foods are richer in nutrients and lower in toxins, more of the good and less of the bad. Win-win. This adds up and makes a big difference in time. Organic is more expensive, and it's important to buy the organic variety of some foods more than others. My general rule of thumb is this—if the food has a hard outer covering that you don't eat—like a banana, cantaloup, or avocado—you can save your money and not buy organic. However, for foods that you eat without removing an outer covering—like berries, leafy greens, and apples—it is worth the extra to splurge for the organic.

There is a great resource called the Environmental Working Group (EWG). The group updates and publishes the "clean 15" and "dirty dozen" each year. The dirty dozen are the 12 most potentially toxic foods that you should always buy organic if possible. The clean 15 are the 15 foods that are generally safe to buy the non-organic version of, so you can save some money here.

Tip 9—Eat before you are starving.

It's so much easier to make a good decision before you are hungry. We want to eat for many reasons. Hunger is just one of them. Having a consistent schedule with what you'll eat and when can help keep you on track. Often at 3 p.m., many people are not very hungry. However, by 4 p.m., just one hour later, you can be tired, hungry, and ready for a break. If you recognize this pattern and choose to make a healthy choice at 3 p.m., you can much more easily combat the urge to binge on sugar at 4 p.m. However, if you choose not to eat, to not take in the calories when you are not even that hungry, frequently by 4 p.m., you are more likely to binge on foods you didn't plan on eating if they are available. It's almost like your willpower goes from good to terrible in a matter of seconds, and sometimes it feels as if you are almost eating against your will.

Tip 10—Have a plan, and stick to it.

This goes along with the above tip. You are setting yourself up for failure if you fail to plan. When the healthy options are there and ready to go and the unhealthy options aren't, you are much more likely to be successful. This isn't hard, it just takes a little forethought. Plan what you are going to eat during the week ahead on the weekend. Buy the food, prepare it, and have it ready to go. Also avoid buying foods that are not in alignment with your overall health goals. If it isn't your pantry, you are less likely to eat it.

This is hard, I know. And the way our brain is wired for survival doesn't make this easy for us. Just like animals, we humans have a primitive part of our brain. This part of the brain is wired for three things:

1. To seek pleasure
2. To avoid pain
3. To exert as little energy as possible

This primitive part of our brain is wired to keep us alive and is focused on the here and now. The primitive brain isn't focused on the long term. Animals don't plan for the future, and your primitive brain doesn't either.

However, while we share some survival instincts with animals, humans also have a more evolved part of the brain called the prefrontal cortex. This is the planning part of the brain. It's in the prefrontal cortex that we can create big dreams and come up with plans and goals for our future. So here's how this plays out. On Sunday, you plan your week—based on your preferences and what you truly want for your health and your life. This all occurs in the evolved part of the brain, the prefrontal cortex. Then by mid-week, as the willpower is getting low, your primitive brain sends you messages like, "This is stupid," "You don't have to follow this plan," "Just this one time won't matter," or my personal favorite, "It's been such a rough day." You can find a reason why you deserve a treat almost every day because it's rare that days go 100 percent according to your plan and preferences. These sneaky little thoughts can cause you to give up at the moment, so you have to be ready for them.

Anticipate these thoughts and have a plan to combat them. Some options are, "Yes, I hear you, brain, and I understand, but I have a plan, and I'm sticking to it." It's the little toddler inside all of us, screaming and throwing a fit for a candy bar at the gas station. If you say no, eventually your brain will quit throwing the fit. But if you say yes—you'll be reinforcing the behavior of your toddler brain, which makes you happy in the moment but keeps you further and further away from your bigger dreams and goals in life. The more you give in to this urge, the stronger it becomes in the future. Just like saying yes to the toddler in the gas station makes it harder to say no the next time since the behavior has previously been reinforced. The good news is that the urge-reward cycle can be deconditioned too.

A Pavlovian response, otherwise known as classical conditioning, is a behavior that occurs when a potent stimulus is paired with a previously neutral stimulus. An example would be desiring a candy bar (potent stimulus) every time you stop at the gas station (neutral stimulus) to fuel your car. This response was first defined in a psychological experiment done by Ivan Pavlov in the late 1800s, where dogs were given food at the same time a bell was rung. Like most dogs, the food alone caused Pavlov's dogs to salivate. After pairing the potent stimulus (food) with the neutral stimulus (bell), eventually ringing the bell alone elicited salivation for these dogs. The dogs quickly learned that when they heard the bell, food was coming, just like we can easily anticipate a treat is coming as we fuel up our car. It doesn't take long for this pairing to happen. However, the good news is, it doesn't take long to uncouple the two stimuli either. Pavlov deconditioned his dogs by ringing the bell and not providing food. Pavlov's dogs eventually quit salivating when the bell was rung and the food was no longer given. You can decondition your brain in the same way by not giving in to these urges you have for treats. Of course, the first time you stop at the gas station and don't indulge in a treat, it will be hard. However, after resisting the urge a few times, it becomes easier and easier, and eventually it isn't even a struggle at all.

We all have a limited amount of willpower and trying to resist temptations by willpower alone works well in the short term, but isn't sustainable. However, if you decondition your desire, you can achieve your goals more easily. Every time you have an urge and don't give in to it, you are strengthening the path you want for your life, committing to your path of intention, the path you chose with your evolved prefrontal cortex. Every time you give in to the urge of your primitive brain, you make the urge stronger. Practice noticing urges and ignoring them. You can do it, and it gets so much easier with time and practice.

NATE'S TAKE: DESIGNING YOUR PLAN

OUT OF THE FIVE FACTORS, NUTRITION IS THE MOST CHALLENGING one to tackle. First off, EVERY individual is different when it comes to how their body processes food. What one person's body may thrive on, another individual may react adversely to. This can be true even if the two individuals are the same age and sex, have a similar health background, and have a nearly identical body composition. There is not a one-size-fits-all approach to nutrition. It is up to us to create our own plan.

Second, our environment sets us up to fail. Drive down main street in any town, and look to your left and right. Pull into any gas station, or walk into any convenient store. The neon lights of temptation are EVERYWHERE. Fast food, energy drinks, sugary snacks, mini-size bottles of alcohol, you name it, they are right at your fingertips, and year by year they are being pushed in your face more and more. Just look at the checkout line at any gas station you now walk into. They have literally lines created by moveable shelves with sugary processed foods.

The third problem that we face as Americans is finding the truth from our "experts" on what a healthy diet is. The USDA has been adopting and suggesting recommendations for healthy eating since 1894, before specific vitamins and minerals had even been discovered. As time went on, recommendations shifted. Below is how the recommendations by the USDA have changed over the last 80 years.

- ☯ The "Basic 7" food guide was developed in 1942, in hopes to maintain nutrition standards during wartime food rationing. The basic seven foods included the following:
    * Green and yellow vegetables
    * Oranges, tomatoes, and grapefruit
    * Potatoes and other vegetables and fruit
    * Milk and milk products
    * Meat, poultry, fish, and eggs
    * Bread, flour, and cereals

* Butter and fortified margarine

- From 1956 to 1992 the USDA recommended its "Basic Four" food groups model of milk, meat, fruit and vegetables, and bread and cereals.

- In 1992 the USDA attached serving recommendations to the new "Food Pyramid," advising Americans to believe that we should be eating 6 to 11 servings of primarily refined grains in bread, cereal, rice, and pasta.

- From 2005 to 2011 the USDA changed the recommendations from the food pyramid to "My Pyramid." This variation incorporates the idea of exercise by creating steps to our pyramid. They excluded the specific serving suggestions and added vertical wedges to give the visual of intake suggestions per each food group.

- Established in 2011, the current food model is known as "My Plate." My Plate includes five food groups, with fruit and vegetables taking up half the plate, half the plate consisting of protein and grains, with a small side of dairy.

Inconsistency on the truth of what a healthy diet is, from 1950 to the present day, has created a real rollercoaster in the health of Americans. Over the course of the last 60 to 70 years, we have seen changes from our supposed "experts" in USDA guidelines on how Americans are supposed to eat five different times. We may be able to remember health class and other commercials that aired during the '80s and '90s that pushed this idea of 6 to 11 servings of grains. Our parents stressed the quantity of food eaten in these groups daily and how it was important to eat them, along with the idea of milk "doing a body good."

So if you are struggling with the temptation of a Pop-Tart, toaster strudel, or any other sugary cereal, realize you are NOT alone. Not only are these treats packed full of sugar, keeping our brains begging for them, but most of us were also raised and being told by trusted adults that this was good for us.

Who do we trust as time passes when it comes to nutrition guidance? The only thing covered above is what was suggested by the USDA. For years large food manufacturing companies have fought for our attention by creating innovative marketing campaigns. Some of these slogans became part of our American culture, like "Have a Coke and a smile," "Where's the beef?" and "Mikey likes it." What actually does a body good? Is it high carb or low carb? Does fat make you fat, or does sugar make you fat? Which fat is good: trans-fat, saturated fat, unsaturated fat, or polyunsaturated fat? And the list goes on and on. If you are looking for diet or nutrition advice out there, which one should you follow?

There are nearly as many diets as there are types of fats. Should you follow the paleo diet, vegan diet, low-carb diet, Atkins diet, ultra-low-fat diet, the Zone Diet, Weight Watchers, Jenny Craig, South Beach diet, Whole 30 diet, or all juice diet? With so many choices out there, it's easy to see why we are always looking for the quick fix. When we aren't seeing quick, easy results on our current plan, we think another one is the answer. Often, we never stick with anything long enough to see meaningful, long-lasting results.

You can walk into almost any workplace across the United States, step into the lunchroom, and find a co-worker who is an "expert" in any one of these diets. It will definitely keep you entertained and maybe even informed. However, it may provide minimal expertise. From milk doing a body good to breakfast being the most important meal of the day and a million other tricks, the food industry over the last hundred years has become somewhat of a bad science experiment that has left millions of unhealthy citizens in its wake.

When it comes to grabbing the attention of the consumer, companies will attempt every trick in the book to get their highest return on investment. No matter the industry, it has come down to how they can get the consumer addicted to buy or use more of a product.

In 1970, the obesity rate in the United States was roughly 15 percent. In 2020, we are fast approaching the 40 percent mark. We have become a society where bigger is better. Why have king-size when you can have family-size? It started with McDonald's "Supersize," and Burger King could not be outdone and went "King-size," and Wendy's left us literally "Biggie Sized" into the late '80s. Although the names have left us, the portion size of that era has not.

Now that we've confirmed (as you probably already expected) that you are the bullseye of every food company out there, how do you protect yourself? How do you make sure you are creating good eating habits, rather than taking advice from these profit-driving companies like General Mills and Coca-Cola? How can you create a nutrition plan that you can stick with long term?

Many of us have white-knuckled through so many 30-day plans we can't even keep track of them anymore. This yo-yo dieting destroys our metabolism. We already have enough working against us when it comes to metabolism as we age.

It isn't your fault. We are all set up to fail, but remember, you have a choice—stay the same, or do something. You are in control of your destiny. If you want something different in life than what everyone else has, you have to do something different. You can be the hero of your own story. So let's find a more intuitive way of eating that you can stick with not just for 30 days, but for life.

RATE YOURSELF AND CREATE A DIET PLAN

Again, you need to start with the four steps just like you did in assessing your sleep.

1. Self-assessment—Where am I currently at?
2. Create a plan—Where am I trying to go?
3. Implementation of plan—Put plan in motion, daily discipline.
4. Tracking—Is my plan working?

STEP 1 EVALUATION

DIET—RATE YOURSELF

Rate yourself from 1   2   3   4   5   6   7   8   9   10

(With 1 being fast food one to two times a day and 10 being real food, nothing processed, perfect portions, seven days a week).

Top 3 foods you love to eat that are nourishing to your body:

_____

_____

_____

Top 3 foods you love to eat that you wish you could resist:

_____

_____

_____

Every time I stop at a gas station, I purchase

_____

Be honest with yourself about the path you are currently on and the journey you'd ideally like to take. Everyone's plan is going to be different based on where you are and where you want to go. An all-pro offensive lineman for the Green Bay Packers probably has a much different plan than the winner of the Boston Marathon. Both of these athletes in their prospective fields are the elite of the elite. Their nutrition plans, however, are significantly different. On average, an offensive lineman in the NFL has a daily calorie intake in the 7,000- to 8,000-calorie mark, much higher than the 2,000 to 2,500 calories the average adult consumes. The expectation of these linemen is to weigh over 300 pounds. It is simple physics: the larger the object, the more difficult it is to move. Now, on the other end of the spectrum, the average marathon runner is somewhere in the 140-pound range, give or take a few pounds. The more muscle, the more weight. The more body fat, the more weight. When you consider the distance they cover and the amount of time it takes them, every ounce counts.

In order to create a plan, you must first identify your goals. Before you can map it out, you need to know where you are going. There are a couple of non-negotiables for overall health and wellness, but for the most part, it depends on your specific goal. We can basically put people into the following three different groups when it comes to nutrition and diet:

1. Weight loss
2. Healthy lifestyle
3. Performance

During different times of our lives, our goals may change. For the offensive lineman, from high school, college, and into the NFL, his eating was solely based on performance. The average career length for an NFL player is 3.3 years. After they finish their professional sports career, they have to find a healthy lifestyle balance that does not consist of eating 8,000 calories a day because they no longer need to keep their weight above 300 pounds. Same idea goes for a mom who was once a high school or college athlete. Just as our body changes as we get older, so does the way that it reacts and processes the foods that we take in.

WEIGHT LOSS

IN ORDER TO LOSE WEIGHT, YOU KNOW THAT IT IS A MATTER OF calories in your body versus the physical output of your body. Many know that a pound of body fat is roughly 3,500 calories, so in order to lose weight, you must keep intake lower in relation to your output or physical exertion. An analogy we can use is one of driving a car. You do not need to fill up the gas tank if you are not going to pull your car out of the garage. So just like a vehicle, you do not need to fill your body with 2, 3, or 4 thousand calories if you are only going to go from bed, to chair, to couch, and back to bed every day. To go along with that comparison, we can also compare the fuel that you put in cars, to the fuel that you put in your belly. The quality of the fuel used translates to both athletic performance and how you feel. You wouldn't fill up your Porsche with the cheapest, lowest octane fuel available and expect it to perform optimally. Yet perhaps you do this with your body and wonder why you aren't feeling great and performing better.

PLANNING FOR WEIGHT LOSS

Level 1—Rating 1–3

If you are in the range of **1 to 3** on your nutrition scale, then you must start simply and not get lost in the gimmicks of losing weight fast. The goal is to build a healthy, sustainable lifestyle that allows for grace during certain times of your life. Just like a real financial investment, the more investing in your health on the front end gives you more metabolic flexibility later in life.

Weeks one and two might include getting rid of—or at least cutting back on—soda and other sugary drinks. If you normally drink a soda with lunch every day, limit it to two times a week. If you eat out for lunch every day, pack something Monday, Wednesday, and Friday, and eat out only on Tuesday and Thursday. When you do eat out, try selecting a healthier option. No matter what plan you have, the key to success is making a plan and sticking to it. If you have planned to not eat out Monday to Friday, then when a co-worker asks you to grab something to eat with them, you must say no. You can answer, "Hey, let me know ahead of time. I plan on grabbing something tomorrow if you want to go." There is a graceful way to do it, but be prepared to take some harassment from friends and co-workers as living a healthy lifestyle and choosing not to hit a happy hour on a Friday after work could make you an outcast in some situations.

The truth is, you want to stick with the plan you create, or you wouldn't have created it in the first place. When temptations arise, it's so easy to just throw the plan out of the window and live in the moment. That is a battle that will never go away. It comes from the primitive brain, which is trying to keep you alive. The idea is that the more you say no, the easier it becomes. Before you know it, you don't even have to think about it, like Pavlov's dogs. You can condition your brain to make this easy. Good habits are hard to start because the rewards aren't immediately evident. The primitive brain is wired to seek comfort and pleasure NOW. Bad habits are so much easier because the payoff is NOW. You get immediate gratification from the pleasure of the food, but this immediate reward keeps you further and further from the long-term goals you have for your health and your life.

Level 2—Rating 4–6

If you are a **4 to 6** on that nutritional scale and you want to improve to a **7 to 10,** what steps can you take? Typically, that answer is to be more disciplined in your decision-making and sharpen your skills when it comes to planning. The first step would be a five-day work week meal prep. You can do this either yourself, or there are many companies out there that can take care of it for you. Some simple planning that would help get you to that next level is having all lunches and snacks pre-planned and portioned. If you can do this for all members of your household, it instantly increases your chance of success. Have them join in cutting, portioning, and weighing the meals and snacks. They can pre-package their own fruits and vegetables for after school or before sporting events. Also, give them a choice in the matter when it comes to what "healthy" foods they are pre-packaging.

The picture is much bigger than what we are planning for next week, next month, or even next year. If we can equip our future generations with knowledge of what health is, and the importance of planning and creating healthy habits, then we are leaving our children much better off than we were at their age. Knowledge is power!

Level 3—Rating 7–10

If you are in the 7 to 10 category, you are ready to level up your nutrition by tracking what you are eating. The little bad decisions here and there will start to add up, and before you know it, your nutrition has fallen off track, and you have put on an additional 10 to 20 pounds. A great way to make sure you stay on track is by calculating your calories and macronutrients. It doesn't matter if your goals are to lose weight, perform, or just maintain a healthy balance; by calculating what goes into your body, you are able to refine and identify how foods make you feel, so you can identify when a change is needed. Remember that when you are eating the right foods, you are able to eat more, but when you are eating the calorie-dense, processed foods, you leave your body hungry for more. It makes sense, those processed foods (even though they taste so darn good) are deplete of the nutrients the body needs.

Macronutrients are the fats, proteins, and carbohydrates that are found in foods. Creating a good ratio between these three in your daily nutrient intake is optimal for overall health and wellness. Depending on your goals, the ratio of macros will vary from person to person. A general guideline for what your diet should consist of is found below.

MACRO COUNTING 101

Carbohydrates—45 to 65 percent of your daily intake

Fats—25 to 35 percent of your daily intake

Protein—10 to 30 percent of your daily intake

Example: 2,000-calorie diet

40 percent carb— 2,000 x 40 percent = 800 calories

30 percent fat—2,000 x 30 percent = 600 calories

30 percent protein—2,000 x 30 percent = 600 calories

Carb 1 gram = 4 calories

Fat 1 gram = 9 calories

Protein 1 gram = 4 calories

To find out how many grams a day you should eat of each, you divide them each by the calorie.

Carb: 800/4 = 200 grams per day

Fat: 600/9 = 66.6 grams per day

Protein: 600/4 = 150 grams per day

If you follow Dr. Libby's Top 10 Tips for Eating Healthy and count your macros seven days a week, you will have mastered dieting and will be well on your way to living your best life.

Here are some great free nutrition trackers to help calculate your macros:

- My Fitness Pal
- Calorie Counter
- FatSecret
- MyPlate Calorie Counter
- NutritionFacts

SIMPLE HACKS ON SUCCESSFUL NUTRITION—TIPS TO KNOW YOUR TRIGGERS

Tip 1—Just say NO at the store.

If you don't buy it, it is easier not to eat it, especially while at home. If I had to go face to face with brown sugar and cinnamon Pop-Tarts every morning, I am 100 percent confident I would lose, especially at first. Walking by them and saying no to them at home is much more difficult than walking by them and saying no in the store. If you don't have potato chips, ice cream, and Fruity Pebbles in the house, you don't have to worry about eating them. The best option is DO NOT buy them so that you do not have them easily accessible to eat. Control your environment.

What about the kids?! What about them? Over time kids will get used to not having chips, fruit snacks, cereal, and other sweet treats. Pop-Tarts and cereal are easy, and that's why we buy them. But let's be honest, it is the lazy thing to do as a parent. You may not believe it, but if you cut up some strawberries or clean some blueberries and leave them sitting out, your children will start to come around to healthier options. We have a society that is addicted to sugar, and that addiction typically starts in childhood. You can stop the addiction before it starts and help them develop positive habits that will follow them into adulthood.

Tip 2—Leave the kids.

If possible, don't take kids with you to the store. "Hey, Mom, can we pick up more of those apples and broccoli, those are my favorite?" said no kid ever. If you can avoid the negative influence of "kid pressure," then it makes sticking to the plan much easier. If you must take them with you, then limit their input before they go into the store. Try to set rules like they can choose one item to add to the cart, and that is it. Over time, your kids will start to understand that you aren't dieting, but this is just how your family eats. Set expectations that chips, candy, and ice cream are for special occasions. The ultimate goal is to help them make better decisions as they grow up and start their own families. You are laying the foundation for healthy generations.

Tip 3—Pre-shop.

If not taking the kids is not an option, or you do not have the willpower in the store, then pre-shop your groceries. As a result of Covid-19, almost every grocery store in America has an online shopping grocery option. If you are going to have the kids with you, then hit the click list or schedule your groceries for delivery. This also helps you to be intentional in your meal plans, helps save money, and eliminates impulse buying when in the store. If you do your grocery shopping in person, DO NOT go to the grocery store hungry. Always eat before you go. Bring a list with you, and stick to the list.

Tip 4—Plan your week.

The real magic to any week starts by having a good plan on Sunday. If you love cooking, this is the time to plan your meals and cook them for the week, especially lunches. It is also good to look at family schedules and kids' practices to have a game plan for dinners before the week starts. Those might be crockpot meals or something that can be cooked in a quick 15 to 20 minutes after getting home late from work, practice, or other family obligations. Try to plan out days where you may eat out. It is just important to know on Thursday you are going to grab something to eat as a family or with the team so that you can plan accordingly.

If you are unsure on how to plan or prepare healthy meals, there are companies out there that can help you. These companies specialize in providing pre-made or easy-to-prepare meals that often work perfectly for lunch or dinner. Many of these companies provide high-quality, nutrient-dense foods in ideal proportions for a healthy, easy, and quick meal. It creates the ease of fast food without the poor nutrition that comes with it.

Tip 5—Limit or eliminate the fast food.

Kids will ask, "I'm starving. Can we just go through the drive-through at [fill in a restaurant]?" The answer is NO. You can say to your child, "You'll be OK. I have dinner ready at home. You can wait 20 minutes until we get there." You will eventually get to the point where kids stop asking because they know what the answer is going to be. The goal is for your kids to understand that yours is *not the family that goes through the drive-through for dinner every night or after practice.* When you start making healthier choices, it starts becoming who you are and not just a diet.

Tip 6—Only shop the outer perimeter.

The outer perimeter of the grocery store is where the real, nutrient-dense food is placed. This is where most produce and meats can be found. If it can sit on a shelf for weeks or even months at a time, and still be edible, then it is probably not good for you. Only choose foods located in the outer perimeter of the grocery store.

Tip 7—Predict the AMBUSH.

The goal is to see the ambush coming and have a plan.

- *Work parties and sweets table.* Have an alternative option. Fruit is sweet; that's your best plan. Build your identity. Become the kind of person who passes on birthday cupcakes—except your own!

- *Busy evening, sports, and practice schedules.* Have a snack ready and a plan for dinner.

- *Staying late at work.* Minimize the damage. Drink water, have fruits and vegetables accessible. Be careful with having almonds, cashews, or any other type of nut for snacking purposes. While they are a healthy fat, they are the easiest to overeat. There are 12 grams of fat in just one ounce of cashews. If the average American is eating 20 to 35 percent of its calories from fat, you should limit your daily intake to just two handfuls of nuts.

☯ *Holidays.* See them coming. Have a plan. Add in more fitness. Pre-eat good foods before going to where bad foods are. Choose a healthier option—smoked turkey over fried turkey—or try to fill up on healthier side dishes such as fruits, vegetables, and salads. Limit the bad—one choice of desert, not sampling all—and limit the portion.

Tip 8—Gas Stations = Early Death

Bob is on soccer duty for the evening and pulls into the gas station to fuel up before heading to the away game. As he pulls in, a barrage of "I'm hungrys" come flying from the back seat along with requests on what to grab quickly while filling up the car.

If you are a parent, you are all too familiar with this scenario. Planning ahead and setting expectations for gas station stops will help to limit disappointment from those little, wonderful co-pilots of yours.

Gas stations used to be just that, gas stations. If you were lucky, while you were filling your tank the attendant might hand you a broomstick with a key on it, so you could walk around the back side of the building and use the restroom. Now gas stations are full-service market places that specialize in giving your family quick and easy access to all kinds of processed and sugar-filled treats. Now they even have the check-out line blocked off with candy, energy drinks, and alcoholic beverages just in case you weren't tempted enough on your walk through the interior of the store.

Solution: fill up the car with gas before heading to practice, so you don't have to say no. Another option is to have healthier snacks ready in the car for the ride, so you can answer with, "You already have something to eat." As parents, we often follow the path of least resistance and give in to the begging and pleading. This is where you have to stay strong and plan your family's path to a healthy lifestyle. It is sad that the new norm of American travel, regardless of the distance of the trip, comes with an electronic device and a bag of something unhealthy. It seems like saying yes to these requests is the most loving thing to do at the moment because it is easy and it brings instant happiness for your kids. But is it?

As Jerzy Gregorek, founder of The Happy Body, a program that has helped thousands of people transform their body, says, "Easy choices, hard Life. Hard choices, easy Life." The little choices you make today give you freedom from chronic disease later. It's these changes that shift your path from autopilot default to intention so that you enjoy optimal health and an amazing life.

DIET AND NUTRITION WITH A FOCUS ON HEALTHY LIFESTYLE

IF YOU ARE WHERE YOU WOULD LIKE TO BE FROM A WEIGHT AND body composition standpoint, then what should the plan be? First off, don't be fooled by the idea that thin automatically means healthy. Just because someone is thin or within the acceptable body mass index doesn't necessarily mean they are healthy. We all know (and secretly hate) those people who have a wonderful metabolism that allows them to shove anything in their face without gaining a pound. However, that unchecked consumption of processed and sugar-packed food can have catastrophic long-term negative effects on that person's health. Weight does not determine our overall health. It is simply one of many indicators that provides us with some guidance in regards to our wellness. If living a healthy life over the long term is our primary goal, then healthy weight loss should be an important secondary goal. To accomplish healthy weight loss, continue to eat a variety of REAL food and keep in mind Dr. Libby's Top 10 Tips for Eating Healthy.

A quote from CrossFit that can serve as a guide on your journey to long-term nutritional health is: "Eat meat and vegetables, nuts and seeds, some fruit, little starch, and no sugar. Keep intake to levels that will support exercise but not body fat." That is about as straightforward as it gets. It emphasizes real food, and only enough of it to support the work your body is doing. End of story. Next time you go to grab something to eat, ask yourself these two important questions:

- Is this real food or processed?
- Do I need this food to support what I am asking my body to do today?

It's that simple. No USDA guideline or PhD in nutrition needed.

PERFORMANCE-BASED NUTRITIONAL CONSIDERATIONS

WHEN PERFORMANCE IS ON THE LINE, IT IS ALL ABOUT WHAT TYPE and how much fuel you are putting in your system. A high-end sports car or motorcycle takes a special high-octane fuel for max performance just like your body does. If you participate in activities that require high levels of physical performance, there are certain things your body needs to ensure that it can adequately function at its peak. Your diet will also determine how your body responds to and recovers from the demands you place on it. If you engage in performance-based physical activities, then counting macros and dialing in your diet is a must. Just like anything else, knowledge is power.

Most of what we do is trial and error. We need to test and journal how we perform in our field of play and then look back and document what we did the day/night before. When it comes to our sleep, exercise, diet, relationships, and mindset, we need to fully know and understand what makes us perform at our best. Once we find the system, we tweak and change it as needed to maximize our output.

Daily Diet Deposits (+)	Daily Diet Withdrawals (–)
Drinking water—100/70 oz.	Drinking soda/pop
Eating fruits and vegetables—1 cup	Eating fast food
Eating fiber—25 grams or more	Ordering out lunch
Preparing your lunch yourself (not eating out)	Eating gas station snacks
Eating dinner with family	Drinking energy drinks
Prepping food with your kids	Forgetting to pack your meal
Fasting—12 hours or more	Eating processed food
Sticking with your plan for the day	Eating sweets

Little things add up in big ways over time. What is one small step you can commit to today and repeat consistently to get you more on the path you want to be on long term? Master this step, then add another. The tortoise wins the race, not the hare. You've got this!

Let's talk all about exercise next. Let's go.

DIET ACTION STEPS

Current Diet Rating is a _____ of 10

Three action steps for improvement are:

1._____

2._____

3._____

CHAPTER SIX

EXERCISE—MOVE WELL, MOVE OFTEN

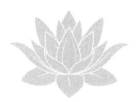

Most people exercise to lose weight. While this is an admirable goal, the benefits of exercise are so much greater than just losing weight. Exercise improves heart health, blood pressure, muscle mass, bone mass, and, yes, it also helps to control weight. It also helps us to burn stress, and if you work out with a group, it is a great way to build positive and supportive connections.

EXERCISE—JAKE AND EMMA

JAKE AND EMMA HAVE BEEN EXERCISING FOR YEARS. OF COURSE, Emma took some time off after the births of each of their children, but once they got the kids on a sleep schedule and established a new normal for the growing family, she got back on her routine. When the kids were too young to be left alone,

Jake and Emma had a tag-team approach. Jake got Tuesday, Thursday, and Saturday mornings. And by "morning," I mean the 5 a.m. to 6:30 a.m. window. Then on Monday, Wednesday, and Friday, it was Emma's turn. Jake usually ran one morning a week and then hit the weights the other two. Emma considered her exercise time her therapy time too. She and her friend, Ellen, who lived about two miles away, would leave their houses at 5 a.m. and run towards each other. They'd meet somewhere in between their two houses (which was always a slightly different spot based on pace and the exact time they left). Then they would run a five-mile loop together before splitting off and heading back to their respective houses to start their day. During these run sessions, they discussed work, kids, husbands, parents, in-laws, schools, religion, and politics. Nothing was off-limits. They got a good workout in and solved the problems of the world. Now that the kids were getting a little older and sleeping during these hours, sometimes Jake and Emma could go to the gym or out for a run together. They took days off now and then—when they felt the tug for some extra sleep, but most weeks this was the routine.

EXERCISE—BOB AND CAROL

Bob and Carol were less structured. Last year, as the new year was approaching, Bob joined a gym. His dad bod was definitely setting in, and come January first, he was going to do something about it. In theory, Carol thought it sounded like a good idea too, but in all seriousness, how were they going to truly pull it off? She decided to see how it would go for Bob, and then she could always join later.

The first Monday in January, the alarm went off at 4:30 a.m. Confused, Bob turned it off and almost fell back to sleep but then remembered, "Today is the day I'm getting back on track with my exercise routine." He got out of bed, slipped on the workout clothes, and headed off to the gym. He jogged on the treadmill, lifted some weights, talked to a few old friends that he saw at the gym, and headed home for a quick shower before work. He decided to sleep in on Tuesday—he didn't want to overdo it. On Wednesday, when the alarm went off, he was so sore! UGH! But he got himself to the gym and did his workout. By Friday he was just too sore and too tired and decided to treat himself to sleeping in. "Well deserved after a busy week," he told himself. This pattern continued for a couple of weeks until their youngest got sick with strep throat. Their sleep was disrupted for a couple of nights, so going to the gym the next day wasn't a priority. This was totally understandable, but unfortunately this was enough to get Bob out of the routine that wasn't yet well enough established, and by the second week of February, he was paying a monthly membership to a gym that he wasn't using at all. "I'll get back at it soon," he thought, but deep down inside, he knew it probably wasn't going to happen. "It'll be easier when the kids are older," he told himself, "One day."

Just like nutrition, exercise is complicated. But do we have to make it as complicated as we do?

THE STANDARD AMERICAN LIFESTYLE—THEN AND NOW

MOST OF OUR PARENTS AND GRANDPARENTS DID NOT SPEND A LOT of time in the gym doing formal exercise. Should they have? Well, with every question we ask in life, in order to properly answer it, we first have to answer the question—what is the goal? In order to accurately assess whether you are on the right track or not, you first have to know where you want to go. If you are satisfied with the status quo and living the standard American life, then following the standard American lifestyle and the standard American diet will allow you to achieve the mediocrity that so many of our friends and neighbors are destined for. You do not need to add formal exercise to your life to travel this path or achieve these results.

Since you are reading this book, it is safe to assume that you are a person who isn't OK with the status quo. You aren't striving for an average lifespan and an average healthspan (the part of your life where you are generally in good health). You aren't OK with just being OK, and you want more for your life. To live your best life with optimal health, exercise is a key ingredient.

Our parents and grandparents had something going for them in their lives that many of us don't. They had a high amount of NEAT. NEAT stands for "non-exercise activity thermogenesis." It is the energy expended for everything you do that is not formal exercise. Basically, it accounts for how active you are. NEAT is how many calories you are burning each day when you aren't formally exercising. What's great about NEAT is that everything counts! Doing housework and yard work; going up and down the steps; doing dishes and laundry; walking the dog; even fidgeting! Some of these household activities can be less bothersome when you remember that you aren't just accomplishing seemingly meaningless tasks, but you are actually burning calories and making deposits in your health bank account.

Our grandfathers were farmers, manual laborers, and skilled tradesmen. They worked long and physically demanding days. In addition to working outside of the home, many of our grandmothers cooked, cleaned, tended the garden, and waited on our grandfathers and visitors relentlessly. They literally never sat down until they tucked themselves into bed each night. Our grandparents spent minimal—if any—time in a gym, but they often maintained ideal body weight and relatively good health because of their high levels of NEAT.

Let's face it, 2022 looks far different from 1950. With the advancement of technology Americans spend more time than ever sitting for work and in their daily lives. Much of our work days consist of long hours sitting at a desk or behind the wheel of a car. Companies take pride in being accessible 24/7 to the consumer, which might be great for customer service, but it has been detrimental to the personal health and wellness of the employee. Fitbits, Apple watches, and other fitness trackers have allowed us to realize that even when we do go to the gym, we often have very low levels of NEAT throughout the day.

Similar to sleep and diet, each individual must build a fitness system that works for them. We all have likes and dislikes, so it's about building a program that works for you based on your interests, goals, and lifestyle. Before diving into the specifics, let's take a look at 10 tips when it comes to exercise.

DR. LIBBY'S TOP 10 EXERCISE TIPS

Tip 1—Ensure you are getting at least 150 minutes per week of moderate-intensity, aerobic exercise or 75 minutes per week of vigorous activity.

This is the recommendation of the American Heart Association. Certainly, this will be much greater for many, but if you aren't here, this is where to start. Moderate intensity exercise can be perceived by noticing that your breath quickens, but you are not out of breath, you develop a light sweat after about 10 minutes, and you can carry on a conversation, but you can't sing. During vigorous activity, your breathing is deep and rapid, you begin sweating after about one minute, and you can't say more than a few words without pausing for breath.

Tip 2—Strength train at least two times per week.

As we age, we lose muscle and bone mass. It's just a fact. To fight this, strength training is crucial. It is recommended by the American Heart Association that you train all major muscle groups two times per week. This can be accomplished using free weights, weight machines, or your body weight. Aim to do a single set of each exercise using a weight or resistance band to tire your muscles after 12 to 15 repetitions.

Tip 3—Get down on the ground, and get back up every single day.

In CrossFit, we call this a burpee. It doesn't have to look like a burpee. It doesn't have to be pretty. But it is essential to be able to get up and down. This seems simple, but if you don't use it, you lose it, and this happens more quickly than you'd think. Unfortunately, there are many people who find themselves in a situation where they physically can't do this. If you talk to any firefighter or paramedic, they will tell you countless stories of being called to people's homes to do nothing more than pick them up off of the floor. It is so much easier to prevent getting to this place than fixing it after it has already happened.

Tip 4—Make it fun!

If you hate running, don't run. If you hate spinning, don't spin. Find something that you actually enjoy doing, and choose that. There are so many options, and there isn't one right answer, so don't force yourself into a mold that someone else has created. Pick something you enjoy and go with that.

Tip 5—Grab a buddy.

Many of us struggle to stay accountable to ourselves. However, when we are scheduled to meet up with a partner or group for a hike, bike ride, or lifting session, we will show up rain or shine to avoid disappointing our friends. If this is you, identify a friend that you can consistently meet and exercise with. (Note: more on this subject in the relationship chapter.) One key aspect to optimal health is becoming a person who honors your commitments, not just to others but to yourself too!

Tip 6—Stretch, stretch, stretch.

It's important to not only get the exercise in but to also take care of your body so it can recover for the next workout. If you want to maintain your mobility as you age, you need to work on it. When you are young, mobility and flexibility are often freebees that requires no attention or work. As you age, they aren't guaranteed!

Tip 7—Start NOW.

There is no need to wait until Monday, the first of the month, or the first of the year. Remember that old Chinese proverb: "The best time to plant a tree was 20 years ago. The second-best time is now." Start today.

Tip 8—Try a Tabata.

This is a great option if you are short on time. High-intensity interval training ("HIIT" for short) is a highly effective way to get maximal results in minimal time. A Tabata workout is a four-minute HIIT workout. You alternate between 20-second intervals of all-out effort, followed by 10 seconds of rest for a total of eight rounds. Of course, do a warm-up first! You can do this type of workout anywhere with no equipment. Just pick an exercise, set a timer, and go. Jumping jacks, air squats, jogging in place, push-ups, sit-ups, planks, or jump rope. You can also add some light weights. The options are endless.

Tip 9—Get outdoors.

Not necessarily every day, but some days it's nice to get out of the house, out of the gym, and get some fresh air. Exercising outdoors will not only enhance your vitamin D production from the natural sun exposure, but also people tend to exercise longer, burn more calories, and it is free!

Tip 10—Schedule rest days.

Too much of anything is not a good thing. Take at least one day off each week to allow your body total rest and recovery. Remember, we are in this not for fast results but for forever results.

If you want optimal health and to truly live your best life, exercise needs to be a regular part of your week. Having a powerful WHY helps with staying motivated long term.

Dr. Libby's "Why" Behind Her Commitment to Exercise

For me, I exercise to strengthen my muscles and bones, reduce my risk of chronic disease, manage stress, increase my confidence, and improve my overall outlook on life. Maintaining my ideal body weight is an added bonus—icing on the cake.

I want to be kicking it well into my 90s. I want to travel the world, maintain my sharpness, and continue helping others (even in retirement). I want to be there for my kids as they begin adulting and raising families of their own. I want to easily be able to get on the ground and play with my future grandkids. I want to be able to get outdoors and hike mountain trails without fear of falling or getting hurt. These are big goals, I know. But these goals keep me motivated when life gets too busy, and it just seems too hard.

One of the keys to accomplishing your exercise goals is to establish a routine. According to James Clear, author of the popular and highly recommended book *Atomic Habits*, it takes anywhere from 18 to 254 days to establish a routine. That can be up to 8.5 months! This is much longer than the typical 30-day challenge, right? As human beings, it is good for us to establish routines. Scheduling set times and frequencies for things like exercise can have major health benefits from a physical and mental standpoint. The consistency of a routine will help you break through plateaus. With time, your weight, blood pressure, and cholesterol will decrease and so will your risk for heart disease and diabetes. Exercise also helps to lower your overall stress levels. So establish a routine that you stick to. Give it some time to really become part of who you are. On weeks that you just "aren't feeling it," remember your WHY. Stay focused on the bigger picture.

If you have a good exercise routine already in place and it's working for you, high five to you, my friend. Keep it up! However, if you are finding that you are no longer seeing the results you're hoping for or find yourself getting bored, then it may be time to shake things up a bit. We need to avoid the tendency to become stuck in a rut when it comes to how we exercise. Also, we need to constantly stimulate our minds and bodies to improve by adding variety to our fitness plans.

VARIETY

WHEN YOU HAVE THE SAME WORKOUT ROUTINE EACH DAY, WEEK, month, etc., it's almost like your body grows accustomed to what you've been doing and doesn't respond to it as well as it once did. The answer is to mix it up to keep your body guessing. Change up whatever you're doing. If you run five days a week, add a couple days of weight training. If you have been focusing on long cardio sessions, add shorter high-intensity interval training to your program. Keep your body guessing, and add something completely new to your routine. New struggles foster new adaptations and create resilience and health.

NON-NEGOTIABLE

JUST LIKE WITH SLEEP AND NUTRITION, SOCIETY SETS US UP FOR failure when it comes to exercise. The job, the kids, meetings, after-school activities, and more all demand so much of our time that while we'd like to fit it in, it often just doesn't happen. The truth is, one day we won't be able to care for those we love the most if we don't take the time to care for ourselves. Self-care isn't selfish. You are worth it, and without intention and planning, it just won't happen. Stay the same, or do something new. Stay on the default path, or venture off on a path of growth and intention. Remember that you aren't like everyone else, and that's a good thing. Treat it like a meeting for work that CANNOT be missed. If you lose your health, you've lost everything. You can't be a great parent, spouse, or employee if you do not have your health.

NATE'S TAKE: DESIGNING YOUR PLAN

AS WITH THE OTHER FACTORS, YOU MUST FIRST DO A SELF-analysis of your fitness. An honest assessment tells you where you currently are, so then you can help create the path for where you want to go. Remember, this is your path, and being proactive and intentional is the key to a long-term life you'll love. Your future self will thank you immensely. The steps again are as follows:

1. Self-assessment—Where am I currently at?
2. Create a plan—Where am I trying to go?
3. Implementation of plan—Put plan in motion, daily discipline.
4. Tracking—Is my plan working?

FITNESS—RATE YOURSELF

Rate yourself from 1   2   3   4   5   6   7   8   9   10
(With 1 being no exercise at all and 10 being two workouts per day, six days per week).

My workouts/practice usually last _____minutes, and I do this _____ times a week. When they are finished, I am exhausted to a level of_____ (0 to 10).

As mentioned before, where you are in terms of your level of fitness will determine the path you will take moving forward with your exercise. We will break it down based on three levels (score of 1–3, score of 4–6, and score of 7–10). Before we break it down, let's cover some basic principles of how we should look at physical fitness.

How is your overall health, and are you even healthy enough to begin an exercise program? If you aren't sure, you should see your primary care, conventional, medical doctor for a physical. The doctor will ask some basic questions, screen you for heart disease, and check your blood pressure, cholesterol, and blood sugar. Then they'll let you know whether or not it is safe to begin an exercise program. Basically, they want to be confident that you are not at immediate risk of dying if you go out for a jog. If you pass, great. You've passed the first level.

The next question to ask is whether you have any chronic diseases, such as hypertension, hyperlipidemia, or diabetes? A physical by your conventional medical doctor can answer these questions as well. Diet and exercise are great treatments for these chronic diseases, but you may additionally need some medications to adequately control them while you are waiting for the effects of lifestyle to take effect.

If you pass this second level, you aren't going to collapse going out for a jog, and you are free of chronic disease. Then, the third level is to look at health optimization. This is where functional medicine can really play a role. Functional medicine looks for markers that become dysregulated before chronic disease develops. In functional medicine, tweaks can be made that not only get you feeling better (from OK to great) but that can also up-level your overall health to prevent the occurrence of chronic diseases in the future.

Every person should be striving for certain physical fitness markers that will help provide them with the level of health necessary to live a long and fulfilling life. Remember, you are not just looking at life expectancy; you are looking for health expectancy. It is important to find a health care provider that understands your goals and can help you along your journey.

The next principle to consider is that strength, mobility, and range of motion disproportionately affect our long-term physical fitness. The typical 2- to 3-year-old child can sit cross-legged or in a full squatting position and hold that with zero issues. As we get older, we move less and, thus, are able to move less. We often use the excuses like, "I just can't move like that anymore" or "I'm not as young as I used to be." Like many other skills in life, with body movements, if we don't use them, we often lose them.

While injuries may limit a person's range of motion, the biggest factors that negatively impact mobility are a sedentary lifestyle and failure to incorporate flexibility into your fitness routine. Additionally, after age 30 the average person will lose three to five percent of their muscle mass per decade. Adding consistent weight training to your fitness program can slow and even reverse this trend. Muscles do not grow or stretch on their own. Any good fitness program must incorporate consistent stretching and weightlifting.

Lastly, your physical fitness routine should be centered around functionality. In life, there are certain things we need to be able to do to function effectively as human beings. This includes being able to perform basic movements like squatting, lunging, hinging, pushing, pulling, pressing, and rotating. These types of movements are important to have in an overall exercise program that will help you reach an ideal level of health and wellness. Below are a few basic physical fitness metrics that every person should strive to be able to complete in order to live a long, fulfilling life.

Exercise	Daily Application-Functionality
Deadlift 1 to 1.5 times your body weight.	Pick up something from off the floor. Kids, groceries, yourself, storage totes, etc.
Squat (all variations) your body weight.	Sitting down and standing up are essential to life.
Overhead press 75 percent of your body weight.	Lifting up kids, putting things on shelves, etc. Shoulder mobility is needed for everyday activities.
Run a 9- to 10-minute mile. Build aerobic capacity.	This builds the capacity for your lungs and heart to function at a high level in all activities. "Aerobic" means oxygen. Your muscles need blood, and your heart makes that happen. Your lungs, meanwhile, become more efficient in delivering oxygen to your blood and removing the carbon dioxide waste.
Complete strict movements such as pull-ups, dips, push-ups with body weight.	Getting up and sitting down to support your body in your daily environment.

Do the indicators above tell you everything from a health and wellness standpoint about a person? Absolutely not. However, this section sets forth a baseline concept for you to measure your health and wellness. The goal is to live a fulfilled life where you can walk, run, jump, climb, and lift until the day that you are no longer here on earth. The five basic exercises above give a starting point on how to measure your level of fitness and truly examine if your fitness will support your desire to live your best life.

Regardless of your current fitness level, you should strive to add in 45 to 60 minutes a week of workout programming that keeps you moving at a high intensity with functional movements. Mix as much variety into your regime as possible to keep your body conditioned and prepared for a multitude of physical challenges. The concept of doing constantly varied, functional movements performed at a high intensity is the foundation for CrossFit and other similarly effective fitness routines.

Below are three workouts that can be completed regardless of your baseline fitness level. The goal is to strengthen muscles and use movements that will translate into functional fitness necessary for real-life living. When two numbers are listed, the first number is applicable to a male athlete doing the workout, and the second number is applicable to a female athlete.

SAMPLE WORKOUT 1

Training Variations—all levels

Functionality—carrying groceries, walking up steps, picking up a heavy box

Movements

Farmer's Carry—hold weight in each hand as you walk

Box Step-Up—step up onto elevated box or step

Dumbbell Deadlifts—lift weights from ground to standing position

Score—for time, as fast as you can complete it

Level 1—Rating 1–3 (160–190 heart rate)

50-meter fast-paced walk

50-meter farmer's carry with 20/10 pounds in each hand

10 box step-ups at 12 inches height

10 dumbbell deadlifts with 20/10 pounds

5 rounds

Level 1—Rating 4–6 (160–190 heart rate)

100-meter run/jog

100-meter farmer's carry with 35/25 pounds in each hand

10 box step-ups at 20/16 inches height (possibly weighted)

10 dumbbell deadlifts with 35/25 pounds

5 rounds

Level 3—Rating 7–10 (160–190 heart rate)

100-meter run, sprinting

100-meter farmer's carry with 50/35 pounds in each hand

10 box step-ups weighted at 24/20 inches height

10 dumbbell deadlifts with 50/35 pounds

5 rounds

The variation on the workouts above is just a small example of how any series of movements can be made scalable to any level of fitness. The goal is to add intensity and variety in your workouts daily.

SAMPLE WORKOUT 2

Training Variation—All levels

Daily Function—putting away Christmas decorations, packing seasonal boxes, squatting

Movements

Bike until you've reached five calories burned on the display for males, four calories for females.

Thruster—full squat into a full pressing motion over head

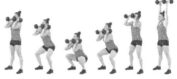

Score—as many rounds as you can complete in three minutes

Level 1—Rating 1–3

5/4 calorie bike

5 thrusters with 20/10-pound dumbbells

Level 2—Rating 4–6

7/5 calorie bike

5 thrusters with 35/25-pound dumbbells

Level 3—Rating 7–10

10/8 calorie bike

5 thrusters with 50/35-pound dumbbells

When we talk about variety, it is not just in the movements that we are completing in our workouts, but also the time in which they are completed. The first workout is somewhere in the 20- to 25-minute range where we are going to be pushing and holding our heart rates in the range of 70 to 80 percent of our maximum capacity. In this second workout, the goal is to see if we can't push our limits to hold in the 80 to 90 percent range at a higher intensity level for a short three-minute time domain. This workout includes adequate rest time between sets to allow for recovery, preparing us to hit it hard again when it's time for the next round.

SAMPLE WORKOUT 3

Training Variations—all levels

Daily Function—trail hike, stairs at a mall or sporting event, walking up a steep hill

Movements

Walking, jogging, climbing

Level 1—Rating 1–3

60-minute trail walk outside in nature, small hills, uneven terrain.

1 to 2 miles covered and 100 to 200 feet of elevation change

Level 2—Rating 4–6

1- to 3-hour trail hike

3 to 5 miles covered and 500- to 1,000-foot elevation change

Level 3—Rating 7–10

5 to 8 hours trail hike (e.g., the Appalachian, Pacific Crest, or Great Divide trail)

6 to 10 miles and 1,500- to 5,000-foot elevation change

Functionality does not change, just the level of difficulty based on a person's physical fitness level and goals they want to accomplish. With the three workouts listed above, you are getting the idea behind the importance of your physical fitness as it applies to everyday activities. There are many different excellent fitness programs out there that can be very beneficial to your health and wellness. It comes down to finding a fitness program that fits your lifestyle and then incorporating it into your everyday life. What makes one better than another? Unfortunately, like everything else, there isn't really a correct answer. The one that is the best is the one that works for you.

You might be a runner or triathlete, a powerlifter, or a yogi. You may enjoy doing HIIT or spinning classes, Zumba, Pilates, and/or CrossFit. You might be an adventure enthusiast that enjoys all things outdoors, no matter if you are on foot, pedaling on two wheels, or twisting a throttle through nature. The more variety of physical activities you enjoy, the higher degree of variability you can add to your program. It doesn't matter if you are in a city or out in the woods, you can always find something to get your heart rate up and endorphins pumping.

SUCCESSFUL EXERCISE ROUTINES USUALLY INCLUDE SOMETHING YOU LOVE

WHEN YOU EXPLORE OUTSIDE OF WHAT YOU TYPICALLY FIND TO be comfortable, you often find something new that you fall in love with. This often is an unintended consequence of adding variety to your workout routine. There are many different great fitness programs and communities out there. You owe it to yourself to try some of these activities. People that are runners LOVE to run. Likewise, triathletes and cyclists LOVE their sports. CrossFitters love them some CrossFit, and they LOVE to talk about it nonstop! Adventure athletes love finding new ways to challenge themselves. Mountain climbing, long rucks, ultra-distance running, and mountain biking are all different ways to explore nature while putting your physical fitness to the test. In many cases, the love for a sport is what drives a person to take better care of their bodies. You want to perform at your best, so taking in the proper foods, getting the proper sleep, and conditioning your body to pursue your passion becomes your objective.

Change Is OK

It's OK to fall out of love with something. As you get older and your life changes with jobs, kids, and financial and social obligations, sometimes fitness goals have to take a back seat. You might be an avid triathlete but also be starting a new season of life that includes a family. The three to four hours of training a day may no longer be your top priority in this season, and that is perfectly fine. Seasons of life will continually change as you age and responsibilities shift, but that does not mean you put your running shoes, weightlifting belt, and whatever competitive gear you once used away or that you put your health and wellness on the back burner. Maybe this season of life includes the availability of 60 minutes a day. What used to be long-distance triathlons is replaced with spinning classes two times a week and doing CrossFit three days a week. Again, the most successful exercise program is one that works for you and your particular stage in life. With intention and planning, there is always something you can do!

Community = Success

Community is a feeling of fellowship with others as a result of sharing common attitudes, interests, and goals. The community can be a physical location, but it doesn't have to be. A community is the group of people that inspire you to push yourself to be the best version of you. It could be a physical location like a gym, an online community like

Peloton, or a group that supports a particular form of exercise like Brazilian jiu-jitsu, CrossFit, or powerlifting. When you are part of a fitness-centered community, you can find healthy activities to participate in no matter where your travels take you. All of these communities share the love and passion for their individual sport as well as a common vernacular and benchmarks that help participants strive for progress. These communities contain the accountability that keeps you pushing forward. It is the person, group of people, and/or the challenge that helps you form the habits you need to be successful in all of life's endeavors.

A supportive community should consist of people who tell you what you need to hear, not what you want to hear. When you are settling for something less than your best effort or selling yourself short, a supportive community will push and encourage you to do better. Too often in today's society people choose the easy road and turn their backs on the road that challenges them with a struggle and discomfort. The truth is that most of the magic in life is found outside of your comfort zone. True growth never really begins until you get to the edge of your comfort zone. When you are constantly growing, you are constantly expanding your comfort zone further and further out. What does your community settle for? More importantly, what does your community allow you to settle for? The next time you walk into a room or log into a virtual session, do an inventory of who is in the room. Is it a group of people that you aspire to be like? Is it a group who is constantly challenging you to be the best version of yourself? Is it a group of people who refuse to be mediocre?

Community is a term that is used loosely, but the meaning is as tight as it gets. Community is the person or group of people that push you to be better in all areas of your life. As a part of the community, you have an obligation to push the other members to be the best they can be in their lives. People are designed by nature to be in tribes. Tribes are communities. Find yours!

They say you are a sum of the top five people you spend the most time with. Exercise is no different. It is important to be in a community that is making you better instead of holding you back, so it's important to pause and ask yourself whether your community holds you accountable or help you make excuses. Do they hold themselves and you to a higher standard when it comes to effort that goes into their workouts and quality of life? Are they open-minded to try something new that might not be what they are "good" at? How varied is your routine? When was the last time you logged more than three or four miles or did some 100-meter sprints or maximum effort lifting? Do you run, ride, swim, and hike short and long distances?

Intensity Gets Results

The secret ingredient to exercise is intensity! Two people could be doing the same 30-minute workout, but how hard individuals push themselves can yield dramatically different results. If two cars leave their house for a 30-minute drive along the same route and one drives at a rate of 100 miles per hour (MPH) and the other at 35 MPH, the final destination each one reaches is going to be dramatically different. On the surface this appears to be a direct result of the different intensity at which each is driving.

However, what if one car is a Ferrari that can run for 30 minutes at 100 MPH with ease? It is running at only 2,500 rotations per minute (RPM) with very little effort. What if the other vehicle is a 1910 Model T, whose top speed is 45 MPH? Running this car at 35 MPH for the same duration of time is equivalent to running at 6,500 RPM. On paper the 30 minutes is 30 minutes, but in reality, it depends on the car you are driving to determine how hard you can push the gas pedal during that time period.

The vehicle you drive every day is your body. You determine the capability of how hard you can drive it. Every day you are either building your engine to do more or tearing it down to do less. It is up to you to find that threshold of building a better engine while being mindful of the negative effects of continually pushing yourself past your threshold.

Challenge Yourself

Consider this. Every once in a while, maybe once a year, mix in something totally different to test your mental and physical fortitude. You could sign up for a demanding race or challenge yourself to something that you have never done. This idea comes from misogi, the Japanese purification process for both the mind and body. It is a notion that has been talked about in books like *The Comfort Crisis* by Michael Easter, as well as on podcasts with entrepreneur and author, Jesse Itzler. Itzler explained, "The notion around the misogi is you do something so hard one time a year that it has an impact on the other 364 days of the year." He continued, "Put one big thing on the calendar that scares you, that you never thought you could do, and go out and do it." The idea is sometimes we can use physical challenges to build our mental fortitude. This concept is also scalable. If you have never run a race before, maybe it is signing up for a five-kilometer race. If you have done a 5K race, maybe it is time to do that half or full marathon. Climb that mountain you've always thought about climbing. Hike that challenging trail that has always been on your mind. Book that whitewater trip that you've talked about doing for years. Signing up for something that you are not quite sure you will succeed at just might be what the doctor ordered for your physical and mental wellbeing.

The list below of possible deposits and withdrawals for exercise includes things that can be done daily. It also includes items that you might attempt or add in throughout a year. Many of these goals will help you plan and create habits to keep you on track. The heart rate zones chart below can give you an idea of where you should be in your workout. Each workout should put you in that 3 to 4 zone and maybe moving up to zone 5 for a small period of time. The goal is to add variety. The more elements of physical fitness, the better!

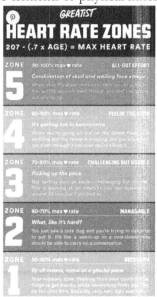

Daily Exercise Deposits	Daily Exercise Withdrawals
Exercising daily—45 to 60 minutes	Taking the elevator
Spinning class	Taking the escalator
Yoga class	Sitting for over an hour
HIIT class	Watching 60+ minutes of TV
CrossFit class	Playing video games
Strength training	Going down a YouTube rabbit hole
Hiking, mountain climbing	Checking social media for 30+ minutes
Walking after lunch	Hitting the snooze button
Fitness competition—lifting, running, CrossFit, Brazilian Jiu-Jitsu	Having friends who don't do fitness
	Making an excuse—too much money, not enough time, too old, a previous injury, not what "I used to be"

Does your path include being able to participate in physical activities, like going on a hike or getting on the ground to play with your grandkids as you get older? No matter where you are currently, there are steps you can take TODAY to move you forward on your path when it comes to exercise and your overall health. Pick one thing. Start today. Repeat tomorrow. Consistency carves canyons. You can do it!

If you are in an exercise community, relationships are an important part of that. Like sleep, diet, and exercise, relationships are also a critical factor to evaluate when assessing overall health. It is often so easy to take those you love the most for granted. Next you are going to learn how to identify and nurture your most meaningful relationships to create deeper connections with your family, friends, and community.

EXERCISE ACTION STEPS

Current Exercise Rating is a _____ of 10

Three action steps for improvement are:

1._____

2._____

3._____

CHAPTER SEVEN

RELATIONSHIPS—INVEST IN YOUR TOP 5

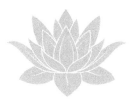

The quality of your life is in direct proportion to the quality of your relationships. Prioritizing relationships with those closest to you and making them truly meaningful is very important to your overall health and wellbeing.

Research shows that human beings are wired to only maintain around five close relationships and about 150 total relationships. The emergence of social media has created chaos in our ability to effectively maintain and manage our relationships. We have drifted away from nurturing our most important relationships and instead focus on accumulating surface friendships or collecting an unending list of social media followers, whose lives seem more interesting than ours. Often, we fool ourselves into believing we have a connection with others because their social media posts allow us a continuous look into their lives as if we were part of their family. Our self-worth diminishes as we compare our lives to the "perfect" lives of our social media "friends."

The sad truth is that many of the people we believe we are connecting with through social media wouldn't recognize us if we passed them on the street. Another sad truth is that we often spend time and energy on our social media pseudo-relationships to the detriment of time and energy we could be spending with our family, friends, or others who should constitute the five closest people in our life. In addition to neglecting our relationships with those around us, we often fail to recognize and nurture a healthy relationship with ourselves. This chapter looks at how we can identify and effectively grow and improve our relationships with the most important people in our lives—our top five. The ability to have healthy and mutually supportive relationships is absolutely critical on our journey to truly live our best life.

RELATIONSHIPS—EMMA, JAKE, BOB, AND CAROL

EMMA AND JAKE HAVE BEEN HAPPILY MARRIED FOR 14 YEARS.

"It's not all rainbows and unicorns," Emma confides to Carol one warm spring Saturday afternoon as the kids are outdoors playing together. "We have our disagreements, for sure, but at the end of the day, we try to give each other grace, recognizing that we are both trying to do our best."

"Yes, but here's the thing," Carol replies. "I don't think Bob is doing his best. I do 90 percent of the work around the house and have a full-time job too. He doesn't seem to appreciate all I do. It seems like we don't connect very often, and at the end of the day when we do have a chance, there isn't really anything to talk about. We are fine, but our relationship is just kind of boring."

"It's easy to get into that rut, for sure," Emma replies. "That is very natural. I think to escape that pattern you need to be intentional. For instance, Jake and I regularly prioritize some quality time together. We try to have a date night once or twice a month. We also, at least a few times a week, put the phones aside and have a meaningful conversation—after the kids are in bed, so there aren't any interruptions."

"That all sounds good," Carol sneers, "but sometimes I just don't feel like it. There are too many other things to do. I think it will be easier when the kids are older and there is more uninterrupted time. One day."

Emma nods in an understanding way and replies, "Don't wait too long, my friend. Relationships need to be tended to, or it can be a slippery slope. Hey, talk soon, I got to run to the grocery and get a few other things done before the sitter comes tonight. Tonight is date night—my pick—we are going to my favorite Italian restaurant and shopping! I went fishing with Jake a few weeks ago, so now it's my turn to choose."

Carol gives Emma a wink, tells her to have fun, and Emma hops in the minivan and heads to the grocery store.

THE LIE

ONE OF THE BIGGEST DREAM STEALERS IS "IT WILL GET EASIER later when the kids are older." The truth is, it gets different but never easier until maybe the kids are grown and gone. Without intention and tending to your marriage, it may be too late by then. We all know the couples who, within a year or two of the youngest child leaving home, end up separated or divorced.

Today's society is a kid-centric society, no doubt. Our parents certainly didn't prioritize our preferences and desires nearly as much as we do for our kids. Our grandparents certainly didn't prioritize our parents' preferences and desires nearly as much as our parents did for us. But one of the very best things we can do for our kids is to maintain a strong marriage. Now, don't get me wrong. It doesn't always work. Sometimes we make a bad choice and we are in a relationship that we can't fix, and the only way forward is out. Assuming this isn't you and you are married to your children's other parent, it's worth working on the relationship. If you are divorced or in a second or third marriage, this applies too. Intentionally focusing on making your marriage great makes a huge difference. This is important to do before problems arise. However, like investing for retirement, it's never too late to start. What often doesn't work is the autopilot default path that Carol and Bob are currently on.

Dr. Libby's Top 10 Tips for Healthy, Meaningful Relationships

Tip 1—Identify your top five relationships.

According to evolutionary psychologist Robin Dunbar, we can maintain 150 relationships. Actually, the number is somewhere between 100 and 250. According to Dunbar, out of these 100 to 250 relationships, we can only really maintain five close relationships. The most important relationship usually should be the one with your intimate partner. But who else is in your top five? Which are your shoulder-to-cry-on friendships? These are the people who will drop everything to support you when needed, and you should do the same for them.

Tip 2—Invest in these top five regularly!

It's not enough just to identify the key players. Don't let the squeaky wheel be the only one to get the grease. Be proactive and intentional about giving your best to the people most important to you. Text messages or social media interaction are not enough. To thrive we need real live human contact. A phone call is so much more intimate than virtual communication, and an in-person encounter is even better. You get out of relationships what you put in them. More on this later.

Tip 3—Prioritize yourself.

In addition to these top five, your relationship with yourself is critical. Your thoughts never stop. You spend the most time of your life with yourself and the "roommate" in your brain. Notice your thoughts. Proactively manage your thoughts. Learn to meet your own needs. This will improve not only your relationship with yourself but your relationship with others too. Just like on an airplane, if the cabin loses pressure, put your own oxygen mask on first, and then help small children. We are so much better at giving love to others when we first learn how to provide it for ourselves.

Tip 4—Read The Five Love Languages by Gary Chapman if you haven't already.

This book can be life-changing. In it, Chapman identifies five primary love languages: (1) words of affirmation, (2) quality time, (3) physical touch, (4) acts of service, and (5) receiving gifts. People vary in how they receive love. Often, you tend to try to provide love in the same way you receive it. However, if—for example—your love language is words of affirmation, but your spouse's primary love language is acts of service, they may not be receiving the love you are giving. It's like you are speaking Chinese to someone who only understands Spanish. The truth is, most people have more than one language, but identifying the love languages of your spouse and kids and others in your top five will help you show them love better. And guess what? When those you love feel love, they like to try to return the favor. It is also important to remember that the people you love aren't mind readers. If you know your love language, share it with those closest to you. It's so much better than dropping subtle—or even not so subtle—hints, hoping they'll get it. You often can identify the love language of those that you love the most, your top five, by reading the book and reflecting. If you aren't sure how they receive love, ask, so you can easily reciprocate love to those you love the most in return.

Tip 5—Don't take those you love the most for granted.

Have you ever been in the following situation? You are in a gloomy mood—it just isn't your day. You find yourself being rather short and snippy with your family—not mean, necessarily, but certainly not overly nice either. Then you run into an acquaintance at the store or gas station, and you smile (for the first time all day), you greet them with enthusiasm and kindness, and you carry on an upbeat five-minute conversation with the mere acquaintance only to get back in the car and resume your gloomy, pessimistic attitude with your family.

If each of us is honest, I think we are all guilty of this one. Why do we do this? Aren't our family members more important to us than an almost stranger? The answer is always—"Yes, but …" For example: "Yes, but … I know my family will love me no matter what," "Yes, but … I know my family will give me grace, and I don't have to put on a show," or "Yes, but … I know my family will always be there for me." This is true and we don't have to hide our true feelings around those we love the most, but I think it's crucial to at least be aware of this tendency, and try our best to minimize our negativity towards our top five.

Tip 6—Forgive easily.

Holding a grudge hurts you more than it hurts the other person. Often, they are living their life unaware of how mad you are about the injustice done to you by them! Quit being a victim, and take control of your thoughts and your life. Recognize that this life is hard, for everyone, even your enemies. Everyone has fears, everyone has insecurities, everyone is trying to find themselves or make their way in the world. Give those who have wronged you grace. Give yourself grace for not giving it to them sooner, and move on. You don't need to tell them, but you can. If you do, you do not need to do it through a big public display or social media post; just forgive in your heart, move on, and let it go. Don't waste any of your precious energy on hate and anger. It isn't worth it.

Tip 7—Limit social media.

One day several years ago, I was at the grocery store getting our groceries for the week. I ran into a Facebook friend in aisle one, right by the baked goods. I can still visualize this today easily. We both glanced at each other, made brief eye contact, and then carried on with our shopping. We didn't really know each other, but we had some mutual friends, which led us to become Facebook friends. I didn't even know her well enough to say hello, which is something I say readily to strangers all the time! Yet I knew a lot about her, and she knew a lot about me. This moment in time changed everything for me. I never feel like I have enough time to do all I want to do, to invest in all the relationships I want to invest in, yet I was consistently finding one to two hours per day to connect with people I didn't really even know on Facebook.

After that day I deleted my Facebook account altogether. I remained off Facebook for over a year, though I did feel out of the loop. This is how people communicate today, so I eventually reactivated my account, but now I make it a point to spend much less time on social media than I did previously. Also, always remember, social media accounts are the highlight reels of people's lives. Your real life (with all the good and all the not-so-good) never will live up to someone else's highlight reel. However, if you compare the two, your real life versus someone else's posted highlight reel, very often it leads to feelings of inadequacy and not-enoughness, which doesn't help nurture your ultra-important relationship with yourself.

I set a timer on my account for 15 minutes and strive to spend no more than that on Facebook per day. This is enough to keep me in the loop about what is going on with my casual acquaintances. It doesn't take much time away from my most important relationships and keeps the feelings of inadequacy at a minimum. Consider doing something similar.

Tip 8—Remember, the kids will grow up and move away.

Depending on your age and stage in life, you may have already learned this lesson. When your kids are really young, the advice is that sometimes the days seem long, but the years go by fast. This couldn't be more true. Being a parent is the most joyous experience of your life and by far the hardest. Your children's dependence will shift as they continue to grow older. Nothing has gone wrong here. This is how it's supposed to work. While it can be sad to think they will move away one day, it truly isn't ideal to have your healthy 30-year-old living in your basement, relying on you for their wants and needs.

When your precious babies grow up and move away, it will be back to where it all started—you and your spouse. At that time, you don't want your spouse to be a stranger or a roommate or a co-parent that you've just tolerated over the last 18 to 21 years. Therefore, take time to invest in the relationship regularly. You should do this to enjoy your life more now and to continue to build a strong foundation for a great relationship where you can enjoy growing old together and supporting each other long after the babies have grown and moved away.

Tip 9—Set boundaries.

Don't just respond to whatever life throws at you. There is often a fine line between helping, supporting, and being there for others, and letting others walk all over you. If you want your life's path to be shaped by purpose and intent, you have to establish some core values for yourself. Boundaries are nothing more than guardrails designed to keep you on your path and headed in the direction you intend to go. Boundaries are actually very natural and easy to develop. When presented with a decision, an opportunity, or a demand on your time, simply ask yourself, "Is this opportunity in alignment with my values for my life?" If the answer is yes, then yes! If the answer is no, then no. The sticky part is the gray area, and if you are anything like most people, there are a lot of things that fall in the gray area.

My favorite thing to say when someone asks me to do something is "Let me think about it." The people-pleaser in most of us wants to say yes to everything. But I always remember this—saying yes to one thing is always saying no to something else. For example, saying yes to the evening community meeting at the school is saying no to dinner at home with the family that night. Saying yes to the extra client that wants to be added on at the end of your schedule is saying no to the time to connect and hear about your kid's day after school.

Please don't misinterpret this concept. You should not always say no to opportunities! Examine each opportunity as it comes. Think about it, and then decide. Say no to the good and yes to the great! If it isn't a "hell, yes" for you, often it should be a "no." Some people won't understand, but that's OK. These are guardrails along your path of intention. It's important to stay on your path. It's the only one leading to where YOU want to go.

Tip 10—Let other people be other people.

We subconsciously have manuals for people in our lives. We know how we'd like other people to behave, so we can feel good and be happy. When they happen to follow these unspoken rules, life is good! When they don't, we often feel frustrated and upset. The funny thing is, we don't even share these imaginary manuals with other people; they are just supposed to KNOW! It's quite funny if you think about it. We all do this to a certain extent, so don't feel bad. The truth is, each of us knows what is best for our own self. Other people know what is best for them. It's not our job to control others so that we can be happy; it's our job to find happiness within ourselves. When we truly find that happiness in ourselves, we are better able to share in happiness with those around us. Finding our own happiness is so freeing because it's available to us at all times, whether or not the other people in our lives are on board.

NATE'S TAKE: DESIGNING YOUR PLAN

PRIORITIZING YOUR RELATIONSHIPS IS NOT EASY. JUST LIKE WITH sleep, diet, and exercise, the world we live in sets us up to fail. Every "like," heart, or emoji on social media provides a dopamine hit to your psyche, which is pulling you away from developing relationships with those who matter the most. Next time you go into a restaurant, bar, sporting event, or social gathering, take a look around and survey how many of those in attendance have their faces buried in their phones. How many people are totally removed from the occasion that they probably scheduled days, weeks, or months in advance? What once used to be a family around a dinner table having conversation about how their day went is now a family eating in different spaces throughout the house, completely checked out from one another.

The Digital Age has taken over, and it has left the skill of developing meaningful relationships in its wake. As the software algorithms improve, our relationships with one another as humans will continue to spiral downward. Ideally this trend will level off in the coming years, but let's be real, humans' ability to self-police is not the greatest. We have been programmed to believe the bigger the better and the more we have the merrier we will be. As more devices are added to our lives, our true understanding of one another seems to shrink by the day.

Most of us can think back on growing up and remember it as a time in our lives when we had some of our most meaningful relationships. We can recall the lessons we learned from parents, co-workers, friends, and teachers. We can reflect on the heart-to-heart conversations we had with those people and how much they shaped our life's journey. Often it wasn't just the words spoken, but the hugs given, the laughs shared, and the tears that fell during those interactions that left such lasting impressions on us. If you think about these experiences and what made them so powerful, you cannot minimize the fact that these interactions typically took place face to face.

In-person experiences have helped us to develop amazing connections to the people we shared them with. Being present with a person and looking at them as we engage in a conversation allows us to fully experience their body language and non-verbal communication. The ability to communicate physically as well as verbally allows us to fully appreciate the emotions connected to a conversation. Nothing can express the care and love a person is verbally communicating to us like a hug that is so tight that we can literally feel their love for us. Conversations through text or social media cannot convey the same level of emotional intensity as a face-to-face conversation. The value of physical presence and the energy associated with it cannot be overstated in developing our relationships.

Relationships are formed in many different ways throughout our lifetime. Our relationship foundation starts at birth to the family we are born into. This often sets the precedence of how we treat one another as we get older. As we progress, we make our own friends in school. We join teams, and often some of our best friends are found in our teammates. As we grow older, we develop romantic relationships, and often around the same time, we come of age to join the workforce and find our first group of co-workers.

The early relationships in our lives are set by default. We usually don't have a choice of who our family is, what neighborhood we live in, or what grade school we attend. The type of people we associate with and how our relationships with these people are formed are chosen for us. This early phase of life requires less effort on our part to nurture, deepen, and grow our relationships. As we pass through adolescence into adulthood, we are often exposed to new people, new communities, and a more diverse work or living environment. These changes will require us to enhance our ability to build and maintain healthy relationships that are beneficial to us and to those with whom we interact. This demands that we be intentional in our efforts to strengthen our relationships and requires us to focus on cultivating several deep or meaningful relationships in our life.

What are the characteristics of that friend that draw you to them? What characteristics within yourself does that friend draw out of you? If you don't have a friend like that, what kind of characteristics would you want that type of friend to have? What traits do you have that would make you that kind of friend for someone else? If you were to do a survey of the people who are most important in your life, what common traits or characteristics do they have? Could you list these common traits on paper? How do you identify the people who mean the most to you? Are you honestly doing your best to provide meaning, depth, and support to the people who mean the most to you? How can you better identify the needs of your closest companions and better fulfill those needs? While you definitely start out in life on the default path and you have no choice in the matter, as is normal for everyone, it doesn't mean you have to stay in that default pattern with all the important relationships in your adult life.

It is important to assess the value of your relationships. Do you have a friend that you could call at 3 a.m., no matter what has happened, and they would be there for you? The relationships between the employees of the company and between the workers and management are strengthened when everyone shares the core values. The same concept is true for your individual or personal relationships. Your strongest relationships are usually with people whom you not only share values with, but also with those whom you communicate with and understand, and whose core values you accept.

1. Self-assessment—Where am I currently at?
2. Create a plan—Where am I trying to go?
3. Implementation of plan—Put plan in motion, daily discipline.
4. Tracking—Is my plan working?

RELATIONSHIPS— RATE YOURSELF

THIS ONE IS A LITTLE TRICKIER THAN THE PREVIOUS THREE factors. It is much more subjective than the others.

Rate yourself from 1   2   3   4   5   6   7   8   9   10

Below are a few examples to help you rate where your current relationships are at.

Level 1—Rating 1–3

- There's no one that you could call if you were in trouble.

- You have no connections with your parents. You have resentment for situations growing up.

- You hate the place you work. You spend more time talking about others than with others. When asked how you are, you answer with the phrase, "Just livin' the dream." You absolutely hate your job.

- You have no significant other, or your partner in the relationship feels more like a roommate than a soulmate. Maybe you've hopped from one romantic relationship to another over the last couple years.

- Most of your social interactions take place online. There are very few face-to-face interactions.

- You spend two to three hours a day on social media or more.

- You with yourself—you feel lost, not really sure where you are at in life, whether it's a job, relationships, or where you are going to be in the future. It scares you, but you are not sure what to do about it. You are just going where society tells you to go.

Level 2—Rating 4–6

- There are a few people you could call, but it depends on the situation and what you did for them last.

- You have connections with your parents, but it is up and down. You go months without talking to them. It feels like more of a task to call and talk than genuine conversation.

- Your work relationships are OK. There are a few people that you don't mind eating lunch with, but that's about it. You might send them a funny meme now and again, but you'd never schedule a vacation with them. It would be miserable to ride in a car with them for three to four hours. You often have a case of the Mondays, meaning you dread going back to work after the weekend.

- You have a significant other and a pretty decent connection with them. It can feel like a rollercoaster of highs and lows at times. Often, you keep to your own spaces at home. You go on dates together maybe one to two times a year, just for dinner. If you had to list three things they value, the most you might guess is one. You're not really sure of their love languages.

- You spend around an hour on social media a day. This is where most of your conversations stem from; for example, "Did you see what [insert name] posted on Instagram today?"

- You with yourself—you have a job, but you are just doing your time. It has its ups and downs, but you feel locked into a relationship or job you cannot leave because of finances or benefits. You're in too deep and are too scared to make a change. You have a pretty good idea of what your dream job would look like, but you are too scared or not sure financially how to make it work. You might say that you are "living the dream," but most of the time you truly mean, "Wow, my life is mundane."

Level 3—Rating 7–10

- You have five top people in your life you could call at any time and in any situation.

- You talk to parents or parental figures once a week just to see how things are going. You visit them multiple times a year with zero expectations.

- You love the people you work with. While you may not be "best friends" with everybody, the culture in your space is amazing. You would try to talk to anyone you care about to come work with you because it's a group of good people.

- About your significant other—you have scheduled time alone time together weekly for lunch, coffee, walks, etc. You know exactly what love languages they speak. You make a point to make sure you are hitting those. You take a few weekends a year to go someplace with just the two of you to enjoy each other's company. There is no one in the world you would rather enjoy life with, for richer or poorer, in sickness and in health. Is this person a companion who walks along with you on your path? You communicate a vision of the future with this person and share a common view of what that future looks like together.

- You might spend 30 minutes a day on social media, looking at posts from friends and family. You might share things going on in your life, but it is not usually the topic of conversations with others. If you did not have social media accounts or if you were never to use them again, it wouldn't bother you a bit.

☯ You with yourself—you are exactly or pretty close to where you want to be in work. You have made some scary changes, but they are putting you closer to truly living your dream. You spend time alone daily, reading, journaling, and reflecting on where you are at currently and what truly makes you happy. You often put these thoughts to actions to help you get closer to staying on your path, creating your own life's journey.

CORE VALUES

So now that you have identified where you are, here are a few action items to consider. We all have an idea of who we are and what is important to us, but how many of us have those non-negotiable characteristics written down? Similarly to how most successful businesses have their core values and mission statements written down, we, as individuals, should also do the same.

The goal is to not just write them out in 30 to 40 minutes just to check the box, but to truly dig deep and reflect on the characteristics that are most important to you. This might be something that takes weeks or even months to create. A few items might change as you get older and your life and priorities shift.

What is the difference between good and great businesses? Good businesses have their core values written down, and once a quarter or year they will revisit those values. Great companies talk and live with their values daily. Their every decision is made with these in mind, big or small. They are the rudder on the boat that guides the company exactly where it would like to go. The core values are not just written; they are lived! Everyone within the organization can share a story about something that has taken place over time in their company that exemplifies their company's values.

Let's dig deep and think about things that have happened in our life and what events stick with us the most. It may have been how a family member treated us, or it may have been the way our mother or father raised us that sticks with us. Remember, relationships are all based on our feelings. The relationships we value the most are largely those in which the other person brings out the best in us. The relationships that are the most toxic in our lives typically lack shared values where one person controls, devalues, or impedes the growth of the other. Whether it's a family member, co-worker, friendship, or romantic relationship, we have the freedom to choose. We can look into our values and ask ourselves, "Am I living my core values, or am I letting others control the rudder on my vessel?"

Core Values—Bob and Jake

Jake pulls into the drive coming home from a morning grocery store run when he sees Bob out in the yard hammering down a sign advertising a garage sale. Jake parks his car, grabs his few items, and wanders over to chat with Bob before heading in.

"Hey, Bob, getting a head start on some spring cleaning?" Jake asks with a chuckle and continues, "I know it probably wouldn't hurt for Emma and me to join in on that one. It's amazing how much stuff you can accumulate in a year."

Bob replies, "Yeah, spring cleaning never hurts, for sure, but we figured it wouldn't hurt to raise some money to help with the mission trip we're going on in a few weeks."

"Oh, wow, I didn't know you guys had plans," Jake curiously replies.

"Well, neither did we, but there's a plan that is bigger than ours out there, and this one is sending us to Venezuela for three weeks."

"Three weeks!" Jake exclaims.

Bob responds, "Yeah, there were some hurricanes that ran through a few villages there, and our church is getting together to help with relief efforts."

"What are you going to do about kids, their school, and your work?" Jake asks.

Bob answered, "I talked to my boss, and he's less than thrilled, so much so that he is only going to let me use a week of my vacation time, considering it is such short notice. We're just going to pull the kids from school and take any school work they have with us."

Jake, shocked and amazed by the news, asks, "Aren't you worried about your work and the kids missing out on schooling?"

Bob responds, "No, not really. I may not be confident about what to eat at dinner every night, but I know when I'm being called to do something of service and faith. It was actually a really easy decision. It will all work out in the end as God intends. It was great catching up with you, Jake. We'll have to get together before we leave. I better get back at it. We have a lot to get ready before we leave next weekend."

ACTION STEP 1

Core Values—Four to five core values that you live by

_____

_____

_____

_____

_____

EXPECTATIONS

ABOVE YOU HAVE LISTED SEVERAL OF YOUR CORE VALUES. DO THE people who are closest to you know those are your core values? If you asked them to list your core values, would their list look like yours? Life is all about expectations. How we communicate and manage our expectations plays a large role in the health of our relationships. Although we may not readily admit it, humans like to receive clearly communicated expectations. It doesn't matter if it is with your child, your spouse, or your co-workers, relationships are easier to manage when each person knows what is expected of them. How many times have you heard, "I wish they would just tell me what they want" or "How was I supposed to know that it would make you upset?"

As a parent or boss, you are responsible for shaping those relationships with your children or your employees. When it comes to other adults, they are free to act as they want to. Your expectations are simply requests that they may or may not choose to honor. The clearer you state your expectations, the better. Other people can't read your mind. Whether someone chooses to honor your expectations for them, or not, you should not base your emotional happiness on whether or not someone honors your expectations for them. You can't control them. You can control yourself.

UNMET EXPECTATIONS

WHAT DO YOU DO WHEN AN EXPECTATION IS NOT MET? HOW DO you handle it when someone you supervise fails to meet an expectation and as a result you lose a client or miss an important deadline? How do you handle the frustration or disappointment when a spouse, family member, or friend doesn't live up to your expectations?

How do you handle it? Which of the following behaviors do you engage in?

- You ignore the issue and hope it goes away.
- You give the offender the "silent treatment" while allowing anger and resentment to build up within you.
- You talk about the offender behind their back.
- You air your grievances on social media for the world to see.
- You call the person out on their shortcomings in front of others.
- You send them a text or write them a note commenting how they failed to meet your expectations.
- You sit down with them individually to discuss the issue and communicate together to help find a solution.

A great quote from Patrick Lencioni's book *The Five Dysfunctions of a Team* that applies in these situations is this: "What tension needs your attention?" As leaders, parents, and friends, we have to face our fears and build the courage necessary to handle uncomfortable conversations when expectations are not met. Remember, courage isn't the absence of fear. It's being afraid and doing it anyway.

We have all been in situations where we can feel the tension and resentment based on something that did or did not happen. It can be with our spouse, friend, parent, or even at work. The longer we let it sit unattended, the bigger the problem becomes. The elephant in the room will eventually come out, whether we want it to or not.

> *The only way to change someone's mind is to connect with them from the heart.*
>
> Rasheed Ogunlaru

SUCCESSFUL STRATEGIES FOR MANAGING EXPECTATIONS

- ☯ Consider perspectives other than yours.
- ☯ Show compassion.
- ☯ Respect one another.
- ☯ Demonstrate consideration.
- ☯ Allow time for the other to talk.
- ☯ Devote time to one another.
- ☯ Set deadlines, where applicable.
- ☯ Set consequences ahead of time, where applicable.
- ☯ Use non-threatening language.

EMOTIONS AND RELATIONSHIPS

PEOPLE FACE CHALLENGES AND UNMET EXPECTATIONS EVERY DAY. Your ability to appropriately manage your emotions in the face of adversity greatly impacts your individual health and the quality of the relationships with those around you. A great quote to apply in your daily life is "It's only a big deal if you make it a big deal." One person can get cut off in traffic and absolutely lose their mind, and another person can get cut off in traffic and not even bat an eye. What's the difference between the two? It's all about each one's reaction to a perceived expectation.

One driver had an expectation on how others should drive, and when that expectation was not met, the reaction was to yell, curse, and slam on the horn, instantly raising their blood pressure. Others handle traffic and the unexpected with a grain of salt. A traffic jam, a flat tire, following a school bus, or another setback is nothing more than the expected situations we deal with when driving a car. There are always going to be unexpected events that happen in life, and it's up to us to see the glass half-full or half-empty. Try approaching situations like this with curiosity instead of anger. It can make a big difference.

In the book *Emotional Intelligence 2.0*, authors Travis Bradberry and Jean Greaves place skill sets for our emotions into two categories: personal competence and social competence. Personal competence is the level of our emotional self-awareness. Self-awareness of emotions is being able to identify the situations that upset us before they even happen. Once we can identify those situations and understand how they affect our emotions, we can then build a level of self-management. Self-management is exactly what it sounds like. When someone pulls out in front of us, do we lose our cool and slam on the horn, or do we hit the brakes and continue on as if nothing big has happened? We understand that we must be alert when we drive because people are going to pull out in front of us. We understand there is going to be slow-moving traffic, so planning to leave early helps eliminate unwanted and expected stressors. To repeat: there are events that will happen to us daily, and it is our responses to those events that determine what the outcome will be in our lives and relationships.

Social competence is very similar to personal competence. Social competence centers around being able to identify with others' emotions in particular situations. People with acute social awareness have the ability to survey a room or interact with others and can identify and relate to what others are thinking and feeling in a given situation. This is what we often see in our work and home relationships. Those with the highest levels of social awareness are able to build the best relationships and are often the best leaders. These are the people that can read a room and make adjustments that address the wants and needs of others in the room. They can see when an individual or team member is struggling and make the adjustment to cater to the needs of the individual members.

It is not the stress that makes us fall, it is how we respond to situations of stress.

Wayde Goodall

Daily Relationship Deposits	Daily Relationship Withdrawals
Calling a parent	Comparing yourself to a neighbor or acquaintance
Doing a lunch date with your child or a family member	Arguing with a co-worker
Expressing your feelings with your spouse constructively	Gossiping about others
Having coffee with a friend	Placing blame on others
Reading at night with your kid	Engaging in any conversation with the question, "Did you see what [person] said (or did)?"
Creating core values with family, spouse, children	Avoiding an uncomfortable conversation
Taking a weekend getaway with a friend or spouse	Lying, cheating, stealing, or engaging in infidelity
Doing a yearly vacation with your spouse	Yelling at someone
Doing monthly dinner dates with your spouse	Participating in negative conversations about people
Doing weekly team meetings at work that cover weekly goals and expectations, especially any that employees create themselves	Arguing on social media

At the end of the day relationships come down to how we make others feel when they are in our presence and how others make us feel when we are with them. Being able to effectively communicate our expectations is the foundation upon which healthy relationships are built. The ability to effectively read and respond to others' emotions while appropriately managing our own emotions is a critical skill for developing deep and meaningful relationships with those we are closest to. If we are not intentional about our relationships, we will end up isolated, unfulfilled, and alone.

The path to maintaining healthy, long-term relationships is not easy. Life sets us up to fail. The easy path is to respond to everything that comes our way without setting boundaries, to hold grudges, to take those we love for granted, and to spend our time judging others' reactions to the obstacles they face. The good news is that it is never too late to become a good communicator or an empathetic friend. Changes can always be made along our journey. The choice is ours. We can stay the same or do something different. The path less followed leads to an amazing treasure of lifelong, healthy, and meaningful relationships. Who are your top five people? Are you investing in them regularly?

After you evaluate where you are in regards to your relationships, let's move on to the last of the five factors—mindset. Life is more about how you respond to circumstances than the circumstances themselves. Nailing this is the key to happiness.

RELATIONSHIP ACTION STEP 2

Current Relationships Rating is a _____ of 10

Three action steps for improvement are:

1._____

2._____

3._____

CHAPTER EIGHT

MINDSET—WAX ON, WAX OFF

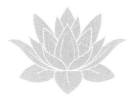

As already mentioned, in this book you're encountering health principles from both CrossFit and functional medicine. According to Ben Bergeron, elite CrossFit coach, the fifth factor of health is mindset. Differing slightly, the Institute of Functional Medicine (IFM), refers to this factor as stress. These two principles are essentially the same, but some distinctions can be made. The truth is, stress cannot be eliminated from life. But learning to manage stress and think about it differently is within our control and has an enormous impact on our health. Managing our thoughts, controlling our stress, and expanding our mindset are all parts of this very important factor of health. That's what we delve into in this chapter.

In the movie *The Karate Kid*, Mr. Miyagi has Daniel do seemingly mundane chores, like waxing his car—wax on, wax off—for a lengthy amount of time before teaching him actual karate. Daniel is frustrated that these chores don't seem to have a clear link to karate. But they do. Not only is Mr. Miyagi teaching Daniel muscle memory that will lead him to much success in the ring, he is also teaching him discipline and strengthening his mindset. Actively working on mindset is critical to optimal health, and although the results may not be immediately obvious to you, you will find—like Daniel did—that investing time here is well worth it.

MINDSET—EMMA, JAKE, BOB, AND CAROL

IN ADDITION TO THEIR MORNING EXERCISE ROUTINE, EMMA AND Jake incorporate mindfulness and growth into their week on a regular basis. Jake has loved to read since he was a small child. He used to get up early on school days to read the newspaper before school, then started reading about American history, and has continued his avid reading into adulthood. He finds it relaxing and loves learning new things.

Emma was later to the game when it came to reading. She used to watch "her shows" on Netflix while Jake read before bed. One year, he got her a book for Christmas that she loved, which led her to pick up another book by the same author that she also really enjoyed. She realized she liked expanding her mind more than watching the trash she was watching on Netflix and even felt like her sleep was improving without the blue light stimulation before bedtime. Now she was hooked. Over the years, the couple has read hundreds of books. Although their tastes are different when it comes to choosing books, they do share some common interests and often listen to an audiobook together on long car trips to spark conversation, expand their minds, and make the time pass more enjoyably.

On top of expanding their knowledge with a regular reading habit and mitigating stress with regular exercise, Jake and Emma also both practice mindfulness. Emma loves to journal. She can solve almost any problem with her journal and pen. Things become so much clearer to her as she writes down things that are troubling her and sorts them out, rather than trying to manage them in her head. She also loves to meditate and spends a few minutes several times a week practicing meditation. "I just feel so calm and so present afterward," she says.

Jake isn't into journaling or meditation. At Emma's urging, he tried it, but it just wasn't for him. He prefers time outdoors. His day job requires sitting at a desk for long hours in an office setting, working his mind. To relax and restore, he loves the peacefulness of the outdoors. On the weekends, he'll often go hunting or fishing. During the week, in the summer, he'll find time to sit outside and read or do some mindless labor outdoors. Being outdoors is so relaxing for Jake, and it makes him feel alive. Often throughout the year, Jake and Emma take walks outside together with no phones or kids. To them it's about enjoying the fresh air, no matter if it is 70 or 17 degrees outside.

Bob brags that he's never read a book. "Why would you read, now that we have TV and YouTube?" he jokes. Carol used to enjoy books as a preteen but hasn't read one in years.

Emma recently asked Carol if she liked to read because she just finished her favorite book of all time and was going to pass it on to Carol. "Reading sounds good in theory," Carol explained, "but there just aren't enough hours in the day."

Like Jake, Bob loves the outdoors, but he prefers sleeping in. He did get up early one Saturday and went hiking in the woods with Jake. It was a really good time. He came home invigorated and excited for life. He told Carol that he'd love to do that more regularly, at least once or twice a month. A couple of years passed since that trip to the woods, and Bob hasn't found the time to go again.

CHRONIC STRESS'S NEGATIVE IMPACT ON HEALTH

YES, I GET IT, LIFE IS BUSY. WHO HAS TIME FOR ALL OF THIS stuff? It's hard, but it is so important for health. The truth is, we are all under constant chronic stress. Failing to proactively manage our stress has a huge impact on our health. Simply put, our adrenals get burned out from the constant demands we place on them each and every day. Our body cannot distinguish the nature of the stress. To our body, it seems as if we are constantly being chased by a tiger, thereby our very survival seems threatened every day. As a result, our adrenal system is perpetually in overdrive. This leads to hormone imbalances, thyroid problems, immune system suppression, and fat storage, and it lays the foundation for both feeling poorly and the initiation of chronic disease. In fact, the effect of stress on our bodies is so common and so disruptive to our overall health that I test the adrenal function in all of my patients in my functional medicine practice at the beginning of our work together. Fixing the adrenals is foundational to feeling great and building optimal health.

DR. LIBBY'S TOP 10 TIPS FOR MANAGING MINDSET

Tip 1—Manage your thoughts.

Approximately 60 thousand thoughts go through your brain each and every day. There is a constant voice in our heads, narrating life for each of us. Some of these thoughts are useful and keep us on track; for example, "After I finish this, I need to remember to return that phone call" or "What are we having for dinner tonight? Do I need to thaw something from the freezer?" Some of these thoughts are positive and uplifting; for example, "That workout felt great. You are crushing it" or "Oh, I love this sweater. I'm so glad I got it, and I feel great wearing it."

However, many of these thoughts are downright mean and unhelpful; for example, "Why is he looking at me that way? He must think I look terrible," "I can't believe I forgot to put the laundry in before I left for work. I'm such an idiot," or "I told myself I was staying away from sweets, and I blew it again. No wonder I'm fat." The inner critic inside of us is real and downright cruel. We think that by being hard on ourselves we'll be motivated to try better and, hence, do better. The truth is, the thoughts we choose to think are optional, so we should practice thinking kind things about ourselves. It makes a big difference. Often, we've thought negative thoughts for so long that without working on it regularly, we automatically default back to our old way of thinking, the negative way. So working on thoughts is definitely not a short-term solution to feeling great. For this to be effective, thought work needs to be done regularly. The first step is awareness and seeing what we are thinking. Then, slowly over time, we can transform the unhelpful thoughts into ones that serve us better.

Tip 2—Read books, and listen to audiobooks and podcasts regularly.

There is so much information available today that it's a shame not to take advantage of it and grow your mind. You're reading this book, so you are heading in the right direction, if not already incorporating it in your daily routine. Mark Twain once said, "A person who won't read has no advantage over one who can't read." The key to creating a reading habit is finding something you enjoy. There are books and podcasts about every imaginable subject. Surely there is something you are interested in learning more about. Instead of watching TV in the evening, try reading a book. Instead of listening to the radio on your commute, try a podcast. Use dead or downtime as a time to expand your mind. It's true, there are only 24 hours in a day. You can't create more time, but you can choose to use your time wisely. Reading improves vocabulary, stimulates the brain, enhances empathy, reduces stress, and lowers blood pressure and heart rate. You learn so much from reading books, and these benefits apply to reading both nonfiction and fiction books.

Tip 3—Meditate.

Meditation activates the parasympathetic nervous system (the rest-and-digest system) and temporarily turns off the sympathetic nervous system (the fight-or-flight response). Many people live in sympathetic overdrive most of the time. Just a few minutes of meditation sends a signal to your adrenal glands (which produce stress hormones) that you aren't actually in danger. This simple technique can have profound effects on your overall health in the long term. There is a Zen proverb that states, "Everyone should sit in meditation for 20 minutes every day. Unless you are too busy—then you should sit for an hour." Anyone too busy to meditate is someone who truly needs it the most. Chronic stress wreaks havoc on the body and sets you up to feel poorly. The effect of chronic stress on the adrenal glands (which produce stress hormones) causes decreased energy, sex hormone imbalances, weight gain, a suppressed immune system, and even thyroid imbalances. Meditation isn't for everyone, so if that is you, don't force it. However, it is critical that you find some activity to send a calming response to your body on a regular basis.

Tip 4—Spend time in solitude.

Do you ever spend time alone? Time on your phone doesn't count as alone time—because you aren't really alone then, are you? You are "connecting" with your virtual world. Sometimes, a break from it all is a good thing. It's good to take a chance to get to know yourself. It may sound silly, but without doing this you don't take the time to know what you want or if you are headed in the direction you want to be headed. According to the wise Cheshire Cat from *Alice in Wonderland*, "If you don't know where you are going, any road will take you there." Take time to get to know yourself. What do you want for your life's journey? What are your values, preferences, desires? Are you intentionally taking steps to live them? It is so important to slow down and think about this from time to time.

Many people take a self-assessment inventory at the end of each year. They evaluate where they are in regards to the things that are the most important in their life. However, you don't need to wait till January 1st to do this. You don't need to wait till the next Monday to do this either. If you haven't done this in a while, do an assessment now. Where are you doing well? Where do you need to focus some attention to improve? Then pick some areas of focus for the upcoming year, and track them. You pay attention to what you track. Take time to evaluate and get to know the person you spend the most time with—yourself.

Tip 5—Pray.

You know that intuitive feeling you get in your gut? I call this my "inner knowing," my "inner wisdom." I used to discount it a lot. Like all the time. I'd look for more rational evidence to base my decisions on. As I've grown older, I've learned to really trust this instinct. It is almost always right. This is a higher spiritual being guiding you. To me, this is God. I pray to God. Then I listen for guidance and direction. Prayer is important. Quieting my mind to listen to the answers that God is giving is an important part of the process too. Instead of just asking for what you need, be still, and listen for the answer. There is a stronger force guiding everything. Harness this energy, and let the power of the universe help you fulfill your deepest, biggest dreams and desires.

Tip 6—Learn.

The human capacity to learn exceeds that of any other animal. Learning is good for your brain. Research has shown that lifelong learning can help preserve memory and serve as protection from the future development of forms of dementia, like Alzheimer's disease. This learning can be from reading books, as mentioned in Tip 2, and it can also occur from documentaries, YouTube videos, and yes, even social media. Is there a skill, a craft, or hobby that you've always been interested in but never taken the time to learn? Learning a new language, taking art or dance classes, or increasing your proficiency on a musical instrument you played when you were young are all great ways to stimulate your brain. Try to make learning fun and to find joy in the process. All work and no play make for a dull life. What is something new you could learn that would be fun?

These last four tips are in alignment with the factors we have already talked about. Don't you love it when you can do one thing and get multiple benefits? Let's explore how the factors previously discussed can have a positive effect on handling stress and expanding your mind.

Tip 7—Eat a healthy snack.

Keeping the blood sugar stable in your body sends a signal to the adrenal glands that all is well. So, yes, snacks can help with the stress response. Avoid highly processed carbohydrates because this leads to a rapid spike in blood sugar, followed by a rapid spike in insulin, which in turn is followed by a blood sugar crash. This process sends a signal to the adrenals that you actually are in danger. However, a snack consisting of lean protein, leafy greens, colorful vegetables, whole grains, low sugar fruits, sea salt, or healthy fats can send a positive health signal to the adrenal glands.

Tip 8—Nap.

Yes, take a nap! Sleep is so good for you. Mediterranean cultures embrace a concept called "biphasic sleep." Individuals living in these societies often sleep for about five hours at night and then take a nap, or siesta, consisting of another two to three hours in the afternoon. This sounds heavenly! It is not yet established if biphasic sleep is better, worse, or about the same as the monophasic sleep that we embrace in our culture (getting all of your sleep in one period—usually at night). However, it is clear that midday napping can promote positive cognitive benefits. If you are sleeping seven to nine hours at night, it is advised to only take a brief nap, or you risk poor sleep later that night. Our natural cortisol rhythm typically makes us tired around 3 p.m. to 4 p.m. each day. Instead of pushing through this period, if your schedule allows, try to take a quick recharging nap. Your adrenal glands and overall health will thank you.

Tip 9—Exercise.

Moderate exercise can have a profoundly positive effect on stress. Exercise increases endorphins in the brain, and endorphins function as the feel-good neurotransmitters. Exercise also takes your mind off worries, improves sleep, boosts energy, and enhances self-image. All good things! Caution: something positive can easily turn into something negative when taken to the extreme. Too much exercise can become stressful to your system. Additionally, it can deplete your body of essential nutrients, suppress your hormone production, and just be too hard on the body physically. More isn't always better. This is where listening to your body comes in. Have a good plan, with a goal and accountability. However, when the plan says one thing and your body is screaming for something else, it is critical that you listen to your body.

Tip 10—Connect.

Connection is critical for optimal health. It is also critical to help mitigate stress. As mentioned in chapter 7, Dr. Chapman's love languages concept can be helpful here. Proactively showing those you love and care about the most by finding their love language and honoring it has many benefits. However, it can be hard to provide all of the connection your spouse and kids need single-handedly. Similarly, it can be hard to get all you need in regards to connection from those that live in your same house.

Brooke Castillo, life coach at The Life Coach School, describes finding a "want match" to meet your needs for connection. A want match is finding someone else who enjoys doing the same thing you enjoy doing. Many of the things you want in life, your spouse will too. This is a win-win. However, there are things that may bring you much joy, but they aren't what your spouse may like to do at all and vice versa. While it's nice to do those things together occasionally, it can be helpful to find someone else who actually enjoys that activity rather than forcing someone you love to do something they don't like to do. For instance, maybe you love going out to breakfast, but your spouse prefers not to. Maybe you can have a monthly breakfast date with a friend who loves that form of connection as much as you do. We are all so unique and created purposefully to be that way. Rather than trying to fit a square peg into a round hole, think about your desires for connection. Look where those needs are already being met, and then develop connections to meet those needs that aren't being met. This is taking control of your life and results in best-life living. You are wired to survive, and meaningful connection is part of the survival process. This is good for your wellbeing and overall health.

NATE'S TAKE: DESIGNING YOUR PLAN

THE MIND IS THE MOST POWERFUL TOOL WE HAVE AS HUMANS. IT is so powerful that those who have mastered control over their minds complete seemingly impossible feats. There is a reason the saying goes "mind, body, and soul" because without the control of our minds, we have nothing.

The mind has done many amazing things over the course of human history. We have created things like electricity, space travel, the internal combustion engine, the printing press, the compass, the smart phone, the internet, email, and—hell—we have even put a man on the moon!

Over the last 150 years of human history, people have repeatedly harnessed the creative power of their minds to do what previously was unthinkable. In the 1870s, the first gasoline stationary engine was created by Carl Benz. The engine produced 0.75 horsepower. It literally was not even as powerful as one horse. Fewer than 100 years later, Neil Armstrong landed on the moon. The rockets that delivered astronauts into space generated almost 40 million horsepower. In the course of a century, engineers, inventors, and scientists were able to use the creative power and discipline of their minds to increase the propulsive power of the mechanical engine by 40 million.

There are also amazing stories of humans who have been able to harness the grit and determination of a strong mindset to push their bodies to unimaginable levels of performance and endurance. Over a 50-day period in 2015, James "The Iron Cowboy" Lawrence, completed 50 Ironman races in 50 different states. For perspective, a single Ironman consists of a 2.4-mile swim, a 112-mile bike, and a 26.2-mile run. Each event is completed back-to-back with only enough of a break to transition out of the clothing and equipment from one event into the clothing and equipment of the next. Completing a single Ironman race takes incredible mental fortitude and mental discipline. James Lawrence did 50 consecutive Ironman races in 50 days. Over that 50-day period he pushed himself through 120 miles of swimming, 5,600 miles of biking, and 1,310 miles of running for a total of 7,030 miles. The shortest distance from the East Coast to West Coast is from Brunswick, Georgia, to San Diego, California. Over his 50 days of racing, James Lawrence covered enough distance to make that trip 2.5 times. Can you imagine how many conversations James had with himself during those 50 days? How much doubt crept into his mind during that period? How much positive self-talk, mental discipline, and goal-oriented mindset work happens when a person is pushing themselves to the edge of their physical limits?

The above stories are examples of people who have a predominantly growth mindset. Carol Dweck's book *Mindset* describes the difference between a growth and fixed mindset. A person with a growth mindset believes that their intelligence and talents are just a starting point, and that their abilities can be enhanced through dedication and hard work. On the other hand, a person with a fixed mindset believes that their talents, personality, and intelligence are fixed and cannot grow. They just are the way they are. These two mindsets exist on a continuum. A person with a predominantly fixed mindset will often only attempt easy tasks that require minimal effort. They give up easily if things don't go according to plan and view failure as permanent. A person with a growth mindset doesn't shy away from challenging tasks, works hard, and views failure as an opportunity to improve. People with a growth mindset look at life as a journey of continual improvement and see obstacles as a chance to experiment and learn.

Where are you when it comes to mindset?

1. Self-assessment—Where am I currently at?
2. Create a plan—Where am I trying to go?
3. Implementation of plan—Put plan in motion, daily discipline.
4. Tracking—Is my plan working?

MINDSET—RATE YOURSELF

DOES YOUR MIND CONTROL YOUR ACTIONS, OR DO YOUR ACTIONS control your mind because there is nothing you cannot accomplish? There are many parallels to relationships that play a huge influence in mindset.

Rate yourself from 1 2 3 4 5 6 7 8 9 10

Below are a few examples to help you rate where your mindset is currently at.

Level 1—Rating 1–3

❧ You believe that there's just not someone out there for you.

❧ You believe that you are always going to live your type of life because your family has for generations.

❧ You have a victim mentality, thinking, "Why me? It's just not fair."

❧ You believe that if you could only catch a break, you could make it out of your financial hole.

❧ You think that maybe if you had a positive adult influence growing up, then things would be better.

❧ "It's just my luck," you frequently think.

❧ You frequently think that if your coach had only given you a chance in school, your life would be different.

❧ You think that your teachers were always awful in school, never giving you the benefit of the doubt.

Level 2—Rating 4–6

❧ Your job is something you once loved, but now it just pays the bills.

❧ You have more cases of the Monday blahs than you would like to recall.

- Your boss is OK, but you could do better if given the opportunity.

- You are in a pretty good relationship, but it could be better. You often settle in your own separate spaces at home instead of spending time together.

- You have an idea of what you would really love to do, but you are too scared to go out on a limb.

- Your job benefits are "too good," so you can't really leave now.

- You can't remember the last time you learned something new.

- You haven't read a book in years.

- You always start a New Year's resolution, but you drop off a month or two in when you catch a winter bug.

- Often in social media you post asking for advice or vent about changes you should make in your life, but you don't follow through in making changes.

- You have a pretty supportive group of family and friends, but all seem to be stuck, idle, complaining about similar things.

- When you have a rough day, your best friend says, "You deserve _____." (You want to avoid people that say you deserve a drink, a piece of cake, or a donut. We want people that will go on a walk with us, work out with us, but not people who will layer on us an unhealthy habit when we are feeling sorry for ourselves or having a bad day.)

- You have general ups and downs, but when you are down, you can be in funk for a month or two at a time.

Level 3—Rating 7–10

- ☯ You have made some pretty scary career changes but couldn't be happier.
- ☯ The people that you surround yourself with lift you up.
- ☯ You catch yourself often reflecting on how you can improve, and you implement those changes regularly.
- ☯ Your people buy you books, not drinks, when you need motivation.
- ☯ There is nothing you cannot accomplish.
- ☯ You know exactly what sets you on fire, and you have created a routine that supports this.
- ☯ You have your down moments, but they usually only last a day or two.
- ☯ The group of people you are around push you to be better.
- ☯ You have never failed, only learned lessons.
- ☯ There is always a silver lining.
- ☯ You view that whatever is happening to you is happening for a specific reason at this exact time.
- ☯ You can reverse engineer any goal you set to be successful.
- ☯ You make a point to encourage those around you to be the best version of themselves that they can.

MINDSET AND ENVIRONMENT

IF YOU WANT TO BE A ROCKET SCIENTIST, HANG AROUND ROCKET scientists. If you want to be a millionaire, read about, listen to, and immerse yourself with people who have achieved financial wealth. If you can find a mentor or a person that has walked the walk and can talk the talk, ask them a million questions. Find people that have been down the road you want to travel, and model your journey after theirs. Learn from their successes and failures. Avoid the mistakes they have made, and emulate their victories.

The first thing I did (and to remind you, this is Nate writing here) when I thought about the idea for this book was send my friend, who had previously written a book, a text in which I politely asked if he had a free hour to chat. I told him I wanted to ask him some questions. That 60-minute meeting started the forward momentum, which resulted in the words you are currently reading.

Secondly, I thought about who has similar values and aspirations as I do. I asked myself, "Who is way smarter than me and also passionate about helping people live a healthy lifestyle?" The light bulb went off, and I sent a text message to Libby. The text led to an in-person conversation, which led to an in-person meeting, and here we are.

The point is that your environment can either lift you up to heights you never thought were reachable, or it can pull you down to depths that are inescapable. The people you choose to surround yourself with will have a profound impact on your mindset. They will either lift you up or pull you down. Unfortunately for many people, it is family that instills or reinforces a negative mindset. If this is your situation, try loving your family members for who they are without participating in their negativity of toxic thought patterns.

Take the time to do an inventory of the overall mindset of the environments where you spend time. What does the water cooler talk sound like at your work? Are the conversations at your home predominantly positive or negative? Eleanor Roosevelt once said, "Great minds discuss ideas, average minds discuss events, and small minds discuss people." If the home, work, or people you spend time with are toxic, then it's time you make some changes.

MINDSET—BOB AND CAROL

AFTER BOB AND HIS FAMILY RETURN HOME FROM THEIR THREE-week mission trip in Venezuela, Bob takes some time to reflect about the trip. The village he visited was physically torn down, but while he was there, he felt so spiritually alive. He had never felt so much hope and love from a group of people, and it now feels as if a magnet is pulling him back. His heart is full of happiness and joy, and he realizes that he hasn't felt like this in a long time. The time his family was able to spend together serving others seemed almost magical. Even though the days were physically exhausting, when he laid down at night with Carol, the feeling of love and happiness he felt for her and their life was something he hadn't felt since the early days of their relationship. The projects that his children participated in while in Venezuela were amazing too. At first there were grumbles from the kids about limited cell phone service, but by the end of the trip, the nightly two to three hours of electronic time was hardly missed. By the time they were packing their things to go home, the kids were begging to stay longer.

After arriving home, Bob wonders what was so different about the people in the village and the culture that made him feel so alive? What was the difference between the people he spent his life with at home and the people he spent the last three weeks with in Venezuela? How could he go back to the office, back to the same ole grind, after experiencing what he now thought life was supposed to be like? How was his day different there than it was at home? Bob doesn't have all the answers, he just knows the feeling there was amazing and he wants more of it.

He reflects further by breaking down his days in Venezuela. Every day the team would meet, assess their progress, and set a goal for the day. They would leave the morning coffee sessions with tasks that needed to be performed by the end of the day to make the team successful. When there was a hiccup in any individual's process, the others would lend a hand to help them out, no matter what. Suddenly, it hit Bob like a ton of bricks. "We were a tribe. We all had tasks for the day, but we all genuinely cared about one another and had no problem giving up some time of our own to help each other out. No one in the group pointed fingers or gossiped about how one person wasn't pulling their own weight." Bob then thinks to himself, "Wow, that's what work is supposed to feel like!"

While on the trip, Bob joked with Carol that he wished they could move their house down to South America. The way they functioned as a family in South America was a complete 180-degree turn from what they had at home. At home he often felt disconnected from both of the kids and Carol. The day-to-day rat race seemed like it left no time to enjoy one another's company. The feeling of disconnectedness as a family at home turned into a feeling of joy and love in South America. It had to be the environment.

Bob can't get this idea out of his head, and a few nights later, he asks Carol, "What if we moved to South America permanently?" Carol gives a quick chuckle, but says, "Well, that would be pretty crazy uprooting our whole family. But to tell you the truth, seeing how happy the kids were at the temporary school and how it has impacted us over the last few weeks, I think I'd be willing to give it a go." She then asks, "Are you really serious?"

"Yes, we can look into it more soon. I really think this could work," Bob replies. He leans over and gives Carol a gentle kiss on the forehead before rolling back over, going deep into thought before falling asleep.

Unfortunately for Bob and Carol, things soon fell back in line with how they were before they left. Though Bob made plans on the plane ride home to get up early and have coffee with Carol each day, like they did in South America, after a few late nights at the office playing catch-up from being gone, those coffee dates quickly got pushed aside for an extra 30 minutes of sleep. After a week or two Carol brings up the proposed move to South America. Bob, who has fallen back into his regular routine, replies, "You know how much work switching jobs and moving to a whole other continent would be?"

Carol starts replying, "I could help—"

Bob quickly interrupts her reply and says, "I think it best if we just stay here. We have too many years in our current jobs to just throw away what we've worked for. Maybe that's something we could do when we retire."

Carol, heartbroken, never brings it up again.

Henry Ford once said, "Coming together is the beginning, keeping together is progress, working together is success."

What Bob realized was that the main thing that was different for their family over those three weeks in Venezuela was the environment that they were in. There was so much positive energy that no one ever thought about giving up despite the challenges they had ahead of them. It felt like the opposite of what he experiences at home in regards to both his job and his family. The energy at Bob's house and at his work is typically negative and reminds him of the crabs in a bucket theory. When you put a bunch of crabs in a bucket, they will try to get out. However, when one crab tries to escape, the other crabs pull it back down. Eventually this leads to the demise of the group collectively. This theory resonates with Bob and his current situation.

The group of people that you surround yourself with determine how far you can go in life. If you surround yourself with negative energy and people with a fixed mindset, you will eventually become one of those people. You will create your own glass ceiling that will limit your human potential. You must be careful when choosing your environment. It shapes who you become. Choose your group of people intentionally to ensure you are forging your path with consideration.

MINDSET AND HABITS

SMALL HABITS CAN LEAD TO BIG CHANGES. FORMER NAVY SEAL Jocko Willink coined the phrase, "Discipline equals freedom." What daily discipline could you add in your routine that would help guide you to a growth mindset? Creating goals with action steps and timelines is the easiest way to get the ball rolling. So many of us get lost in the big picture that it keeps us from doing the small things. Ancient Chinese philosopher Lao Tzu said, "A journey of a thousand miles starts with the first small step." It is important to remember that if you stay focused on the small tasks in front of you, the big picture will take care of itself. Ask yourself, "What can I do right now to move myself forward?"

Are you tracking your deposits and withdrawals yet? For amazing health, not every step needs to be forward, but you do need to have more steps forward than backwards. We pay attention to what we track. Please go to www.thepathofintention.com to download a free companion tracker guide to start tracking the five modifiable lifestyle factors today.

Daily Mindset Deposits (+)	Daily Mindset Withdrawals (−)
Reading about 10 pages every day	Mindlessly watching TV or scrolling the internet
Engaging in positive self-talk	Complaining
Meditating	Making excuses
Setting goals weekly	Arguing about religion and politics with people
Joining a positive community	Hiding from challenges
Doing social media for 30 minutes or less daily	Ignoring feedback
Seeking challenges	Living in constant comfort
Meeting with a mentor or role model	Staying in a miserable job
Seeking feedback from others	Comparing yourself to others
Seeking change	Hiding flaws from others
Creating a vision board	Telling yourself, "I'm just not smart."
Maintaining an attitude of "I just haven't learned it YET."	Engaging in negative self-talk

STAY THE SAME, OR DO SOMETHING

LIKE WITH THE OTHER FACTORS, YOU HAVE A CHOICE TO TAKE the action necessary to improve your mindset. Stay the same, or do something. Be encouraged to take the path less traveled. This is the path of intention where you create your ideal life on purpose instead of reacting to whatever comes your way. Change is uncomfortable. Staying the same and living with anxiety, a lack of fulfillment, and poor health becomes more uncomfortable in the long run. Don't shy away from the discomfort. Embrace it. Lean into it. Managing your mindset is one of the keys to a prosperous and healthy life, and it is within your control. What are you doing to manage your mind? Pick one thing that sounds enticing to you. Rinse, repeat, and reap the rewards in time. Small, consistent actions build up over time to yield huge benefits and lead to what we talk about next—the ripple effect.

Current Mindset Rating is a _____ of 10

Three action steps for improvement are:

1._____

2._____

3._____

CHAPTER NINE

THE RIPPLE EFFECT

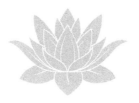

S mall, consistent actions build up over time to yield huge results. This is true with all of the modifiable lifestyle factors. Every single good decision you make in regards to sleep, diet, exercise, relationships, and mindset is a deposit in your optimal health account. An optimal health account is a bank account of sorts. You can make deposits, you can make withdrawals, but if you spend more than you deposit, you end up with poor health. But on the other hand, if you make more deposits than withdrawals, then you are on the path to true health in all areas of your life. Of course, if you only make deposits and never make withdrawals, you get there faster, right? However, this isn't practical or sustainable. We are talking about forever change here, and it doesn't have to be fast. With more deposits than withdrawals you are moving in the right direction.

If you had the choice of one cent doubled every day for 30 days OR one million dollars, which would you choose? No cheating by using Google or even a calculator. At first glance, the answer appears obvious, you take the million dollars. But with a question like this, when the answer seems so clear, you always know there must be a trick. The answer can't be that apparent. If you are skeptical, you are right. One penny doubled every day for 30 days turns out to be over 5 million dollars. Isn't that astounding? This is the compound effect, and it is true for your health too.

When you start implementing lifestyle changes, it often doesn't seem like much in the beginning. Like the penny—one cent, two cents, four cents, eight cents—it seems as if you are getting nowhere! But when you don't give up, when you keep going, keep depositing, keep trusting the process, it eventually works. You have to stick with it. By day 18 the penny is worth $1,310.72. OK, we are starting to see some traction, but we certainly aren't ready to quit our day job with that kind of money. But if you don't give up and keep going, by day 27 you are at over half a million, and by day 30, it's over 5 million dollars.

Some of these lifestyle changes take more than 30 days to really see the benefit, but you get the point. This is the long game. It's like saving for retirement. Starting as early as possible is the best bet. But later is always better than never, and it's never too late. This is the ripple effect. The ripple effect is the continuing and multiplying of the results of an event or action, and it is huge!

DR. LIBBY'S TOP 10 TIPS ABOUT THE CASCADING EFFECT OF LIFESTYLE CHANGES

Tip 1—Creating one small change in your life sparks change in other areas.

Negative choices beget more negative choices, but positive choices propel momentum for more positive choices. When I'm eating well, I'm more inclined to exercise. When I'm exercising, I'm less likely to drink alcohol, which then positively impacts my sleep. When my sleep is good, I'm nicer to my family, which improves my relationships, and when my relationships are doing well, my stress is lower. See how this cascading effect works?

Tip 2—When things are going well in your life, you are a role model to others.

Sometimes the most important way you can impact others is not by what you say but by what you do. No one likes to be lectured to, but people are always watching. You can lead others by example. If your actions spark change in one other person, and that person sparks change in another person, things can compound exponentially pretty quickly. You can change people's lives by just being an amazing example, without saying one single word.

Tip 3—Little eyes are watching.

When my kids were little, my career was pretty demanding. I had the classic mom guilt—always worrying I wasn't doing anything well enough. I felt stretched pretty thin. Years ago, in reading *Freakonomics* by Steven Levitt, I felt comforted to learn that "what matters in parenting is who the parents are, not what they do." It's not what you preach that matters; it's what you practice. Just as your co-workers and friends are watching, your kids are as well. Creating health for yourself creates health for them too.

Tip 4—Your self-talk improves.

Often around the Christmas holiday, I take some time off from my great lifestyle habits. It feels nice initially to eat whatever I want, only exercise if I feel like it, and just live in the moment. While I do think it's important to indulge from time to time, my self-talk during times like this isn't great. My default thoughts are things like, "You are blowing it," "I can't believe you don't have more willpower," and "I thought by now you'd be better than this." I could go on, but you get the idea. When I'm doing a great job and taking care of myself, my self-talk changes to a much more positive inner dialogue: "You are crushing it," "This is working," and "I'm so proud of you." When I pull it back together, at the start of the New Year, the self-talk makes me feel better more quickly than the actual diet and exercise do. The truth is, with intentionality and hard work, we can change those negative thoughts without changing our modifiable lifestyle factors, like diet and exercise.

Tip 5—Confidence improves.

Let's face it, when you are taking care of yourself, you start to feel more comfortable in your own skin. This confidence spills over into other areas of your life. Job, family, and the quality of your relationships all improve when your confidence improves. I'm not talking about arrogance; that's different and unattractive. But confidence feels good and looks good too.

Tip 6—You start to believe, "What if I can?"

As you change your lifestyle and your confidence improves, you start to believe things are possible that you never previously thought were possible. You start to dream bigger. You come out of your cave, and you try something new that you would have never dared to do before. It may work, it may not, but you're willing to give it a try. This can be incredibly exciting. You also learn not to give up. Instead, you simply adjust, try again, and keep repeating the process until it does work. You only fail if you quit.

Tip 7—Life becomes full of possibilities.

When you invest in your health and make deposits regularly, you begin to view your future as bright and full of options. You aren't limited by sickness, disability, and doubt. You can climb the mountain. You can hike the trail. You can travel without having to plan your trip around doctors' appointments. You can get on the ground and play with your grandkids. You have choices.

Tip 8—Your happiness increases because your best years aren't behind you.

Wisdom comes with experience. Life would be easier if, as a teen, we could just accept all the lessons our parents try to teach us, but it doesn't usually work that way. There are many things in life we just have to learn for ourselves. It takes 40 years to get 40 years of experience. There are no shortcuts for that. But if we still have our health into our sixties, seventies, and beyond, we have the benefit of both physical health and wisdom. That is truly best-life living.

Tip 9—A longer healthspan gives you more opportunities to leave a legacy.

More healthy years give you more opportunities to change the world. To be remembered. To do something meaningful. To touch more people's lives. Not everyone wants to add years to their lives, especially if that means living in a nursing home, unable to care for themselves. But who doesn't want more healthy years?

Tip 10—You take care of others better when you are in a good place yourself. Hands down.

It may seem difficult to make deposits in your own health when you are busy in life. But when you are in the busy years of parenting, your kids need you. But they also will need you and want to have you around in the years to come too. It seems that there will be plenty of time to work on that in the future. This isn't guaranteed. Make the deposits now. Your future self will thank you.

NATE'S TAKE: DESIGNING YOUR PLAN

NOTHING WE HAVE SUGGESTED IN THIS BOOK IS EASY. THE default path is the path Bob and Carol take. They mean well, they really do, but life gets in the way. If this is you, it isn't your fault. The default path is the one that most people are on. Beating yourself up doesn't do any good at all. Please don't spend time thinking that you should have done this differently or that it is too late to jump on board. It isn't too late. Begin with one small change today, repeat it tomorrow. Once you master it, pick another, and then another. See the ripple effect in your life and in the lives of others.

In life, we are either in survival mode or thriving mode. When we are under constant chronic stress, we are just surviving. All we can focus on is doing the next thing. Oftentimes in this mode we want to do better, but we just can't. This is where we tell ourselves, like Bob and Carol, "One day ..." Survival mode is helpful if we are truly in danger of dying. If a tiger is chasing us and trying to eat us, we certainly want the fight-or-flight response to kick in and save our life. But when the stress isn't life-threatening danger, this response isn't helpful. When we can calm our nervous system enough to get out of this survival mode, we can really thrive. Sometimes all it takes is one small step and time to compound the effects to start to shift from survive mode to thrive mode.

So what is your optimal, purposeful journey? What path do you want for your life? This has nothing to do with what your neighbor wants for their life or what others want for your life. You get to decide for yourself, and then you get to steer your ship in that direction. Don't be like most people, aimlessly responding to whatever comes their way. You have to know where you are going in order to get there. Figure out where you are going and start taking steps to get there.

Every night before you go to bed, you can decide for yourself—

Tomorrow for my diet, I am going to

_____

Tomorrow for exercise, I am going to

_____

Tomorrow for better sleep, I am going to

_____

Tomorrow for better relationships, I am going to

_____

Tomorrow for my mind, I am going to

_____

Fulfillment is behind intention and discipline.

Make the list. Do the list. Reflect on the list. Does it make you feel better? If yes, do it more. If no, make small changes, but keep going. It takes time. It's that simple … It takes ACTION! So get started.

CHAPTER TEN

ASSESS, PLAN, EXECUTE, EVALUATE, REPEAT

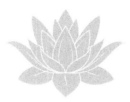

L et me tell you about a wise, older woman that I go to regularly for advice, whom I really admire. She has shoulder-length, gray, wavy hair and fashionable glasses. She lives in a quaint, whimsical cottage not too far from the beach in South Carolina. She starts her day each morning with a cup of black coffee, an oversized sweatshirt atop her PJs, and a book on her front porch swing. Then she takes a long walk alone. She loves starting her day with nature and her thoughts.

She often spends her afternoons at the beach with her husband of 60-plus years, who is still her best friend after all of this time. Sometimes he chooses to go fishing instead. On those days she plays cards with her girlfriends, and they laugh, share stories, and playfully joke around. Whomever she chooses to spend her time with, she is engaged and in the present moment. Whether it's at the beach with her husband or playing games with her girlfriends, she leaves her cell phone at home. She prefers not to be distracted, so she can truly enjoy each moment, and anything else can wait a couple of hours.

Her two daughters have families of their own and live nearby. She talks to her girls almost daily and visits them regularly. She is proud of the independent and grounded women they have become. She has a special bond with each of her grandkids, loves hearing about all of their adventures, and even joins them sometimes.

She has learned that relationships with a few people in her life are the most important thing and values these over things, accomplishments, and popularity.

You can't help but feel calm when you are around her. She exudes peacefulness. She is structured in her routines yet remains undisturbed when her routines get disrupted.

She is almost always kind to herself and others too. She gives herself grace when needed, savors joy, and prays through sadness and anger. Her years have taught her that time lessens pain.

In the evenings she and her husband prepare a healthy dinner together often with fresh vegetables and herbs from their garden in the backyard. They share their stories of the day, then spend their evenings with either a book, a walk, a movie, or friends, before turning in for the night to repeat the same adventure the next day.

They are both in excellent health and are thankful that they took care of themselves in their younger years, so they can enjoy their retirement years. It was not always easy to delay gratification, but they usually did, recognizing the importance of each and every decision. The long hours in their careers and the proactive approach to their health through diet, exercise, sleep, mindfulness, and spiritual connection have surely paid off, and for that, they are truly grateful.

The woman is me, Libby Wilson, as I envision myself in the future at age 85.

I go to this woman, this future me, for advice. She tells me not to sweat the small stuff. She reminds me that the little things I do matter, even when it seems like they don't, and that life gets more and more amazing each and every year. She realized along the way that the journey itself is the fun part. The destination is not static and is just an added bonus.

NATE'S TAKE: HIS FUTURE SELF

EVERY MORNING IS NEARLY THE SAME. IT STARTS WITH WHAT used to be a 5 a.m. alarm clock, but over the years has turned into a little before 6 a.m. on his internal alarm clock. First comes a cup of coffee, often followed by a pretty intense workout that is constantly varied. Sometimes it's a group class, other times it's a long heavy ruck on his own. No matter what it is, his thoughts are often the same, "What can I do today to make myself and others around me a little bit better?"

At this point there isn't much more to prove in life other than proving to himself that he is giving his best effort, as he is his toughest critic. He has gotten much better over the years and gives himself grace, but the thought of a challenge never goes away. After fitness time, it's relaxation and reading followed by coffee with his wife of 50-plus years.

They travel to someplace new every 30 days or so, just to enjoy what the world has to offer. Sometimes it's 100 miles away, other times it's 10,000 miles. Either way, it's never too long as the lack of routine can make him uncomfortable and a bit antsy, even in his old age. They live in a small farmhouse with a large pond and a few hundred acres of land where they can enjoy the outdoors and time with their daughters and their grandkids who don't live far away.

In life he has learned that there is no better teacher than experience itself. As he sees things, while there are millions of books written by some of the most accomplished people in the world, those are nothing more than starting points to guide people on their own journeys.

He enjoys riding anything motorized, yard work, building things, and gardening, as they give him a sense of thrill, accomplishment, and responsibility. Much of the food that is grown at their home is served on their table at every meal. He spends his afternoons chatting with younger and older friends, talking about life, and sharing experiences on how to help improve the lives of others.

He and his wife love adventure and living life to its fullest. While age is a number that often can slow people's lives down, they have made plenty of deposits into their health and wellness bank account over the past 60 years to not let age slow them down much. They love life and their shared companionship.

This man is me, Nate Long, at the age of 80.

Your turn—where are you going? It's an important point to ponder. Spend some time visualizing where exactly you are headed. The clearer you can be on this, the better. This is your destination, and it will help you stay focused and intentional on your unique path. It's equivalent to plugging the exact coordinates into your GPS.

WHATEVER HAPPENED TO JAKE, EMMA, BOB, AND CAROL?

ARE YOU CURIOUS ABOUT WHERE JAKE, EMMA, BOB, AND CAROL ended up? You probably have some pretty good guesses, but let's take a look at their lives, 50 years into the future. They should be well into their eighties now. Let's take a peek.

Bob and Carol worked together to be the best parents they could be to their kids. The kids rarely went without anything they truly wanted and were their most important consideration. Bob and Carol always made sure they had nice things and were able to participate in all the activities they wanted to. They wanted to prioritize their marriage and their health, they really did, but it just always seemed like there were never enough hours in the day to do so. By the time the youngest left for college, Bob and Carol felt like they barely knew each other at all. Carol frequently asked herself, "How can I live with someone for all of these years, yet feel like they are a total stranger?" Bob secretly felt it too but brushed it aside.

It wasn't long after the youngest left for college that Carol went away on a routine business trip. Everyone went out for drinks after a long day of meetings, and Carol developed a connection with one of her co-workers. She didn't mean for it to happen. She was just so depleted emotionally and was longing for connection. Within a year, she and Bob divorced, and she remarried the following summer.

The divorce crushed Bob. Prior to Carol leaving he didn't feel much connection either, but he was confident now that they had time, they could rebuild their relationship and reconnect as a couple. He never really recovered from the divorce, honestly. He began drinking more, entered the single adult party scene, prioritized his health even less than before, and secretly blamed Carol for all his woes. He never remarried and died alone at age 64 from a massive heart attack.

Carol just knew the grass would be greener in this new relationship with her soulmate. In her mind, her only problem for all those years had been Bob. If she had just picked the right man from the beginning, life would have been better. However, the new marriage had different, unforeseen problems. Being a step-parent was harder than either Carol or her new husband anticipated. Some things were better in her new marriage, but many things were worse. There was added financial strain that came from the two households, which led to constant arguments and fights. Carol did have more time for herself now, so she began an exercise program. She'd gone down this road multiple times in the past, but something always came up with the kids, which derailed her progress. This time she'd make it work. She no longer had lack of time as an excuse, but she found it very hard to keep up. Her joints ached so badly after an exercise class that it took her days to recover. This kept her from going to the gym as much as she'd like to. One day she went on a hike with one of her adult children and grandkids. She was so excited to spend the day with them at a nature preserve a few hours away. The hike was more treacherous than she'd expected and nearly killed her. She couldn't keep up and didn't realize all the twists and turns and elevation changes she'd have to navigate. She made it but swore she'd never do that again unless she lost a considerable amount of weight. She had 70 pounds to lose (it had just gradually built up over the years), but the problem was that exercise was so hard on her body. How in the world would she do it? She tried for a few weeks to modify her diet but gave up (as she had many times before) when the results on the scale didn't match the results of her efforts. At age 69, Carol began to show signs of dementia. At age 71, her husband and family could no longer take care of her. She spent the last three years of her life in the nursing home with debilitating arthritis and Alzheimer's disease. Carol died at the age of 74.

Jake and Emma live in an active retirement community in the South. Three days a week they play pickleball together. They are quite a team and tough to beat. Jake is in a few men's clubs, and Emma enjoys the walking club and playing bridge. Their relationship is better than ever, and they have maintained their best friend status, even after all of these years. Their kids are all grown now, and their grandkids are starting lives of their own. They travel to visit the kids several times a year, and, of course, the kids come to visit too.

Their good health provides them with so much freedom. They are both in their eighties now, and, of course, they no longer feel like they are 40, but they take their vitamins, are on minimal prescription meds, and get around much better than their friends even 10 to 15 years younger than they are. They prioritize high-quality healthy foods, a good night's sleep, and mindfulness, just as they did when they were younger.

People they meet are astounded at their age and ask for their secrets. "What's the quick fix?" they ask. Emma and Jake look at one another lovingly and smile. "More deposits than withdrawals," responds Jake. This usually sparks a look of confusion. Jake understands that if they haven't gotten it by now, they probably won't, but who knows? So, he elaborates, "Well, there is no quick fix. Sure would be nice if there was. But years ago, decades ago, Emma and I decided what was important to us in our lives. We figured out our core values, and we've been investing in those values regularly, almost daily, since then. We knew where we wanted our journey to take us and stayed on the path to get us there. We didn't notice any results at first, but over time, well, it's been incredible." With that, Jake gives Emma a wink, grabs her hand, and they head towards home. Jake and Emma got it. The secret to a great life was to have a series of great days.

The lives of Bob, Carol, Jake, and Emma seemed so similar in the neighborhood all those years ago. It really didn't seem like the little decisions would make that much of a difference, but with the compounding effect of time, their lives ended up in drastically different places.

How can you ensure your life ends up like Jake and Emma's instead of Bob and Carol's?

DR. LIBBY'S TOP 10 TIPS TO ENSURE YOU ENJOY THE MOST ABUNDANT LIFE AND THE LONGEST HEALTHSPAN POSSIBLE

Tip 1—Decide.

This is the first step. Are you going to stay the same or do something different? You have to take the first step down a new path to get to a new destination. First of all, decide which path you'll take—intentional or autopilot default. Not deciding is deciding to take the autopilot default path, like Bob and Carol.

Tip 2—Commit.

Actions speak louder than words. In all honesty, Bob and Carol decided many times to do things differently, but they didn't commit, so when things came up, the plans went out the window. Are you interested in increasing your healthspan, or are you committed? Here's the difference that I learned from life coach Jody Moore. When your kids are young and need to be picked up from school or sports practice, you're committed to doing it. You'll be there no matter what. If an emergency arises and you can't make it, you'll call in the grandparents, a neighbor, or a friend, but no matter what, someone will be there. Every time. That's commitment.

Being interested in something, looks more like this— you decide you'll get up an hour early and work out tomorrow. Then, the dog gets up in the middle of the night and needs to go out. This disrupts your sleep enough that you struggle to fall back to sleep and toss and turn. When the alarm goes off, you turn it off and say to yourself, "Maybe tomorrow." That's being interested, not committed. You'll never not pick up your kids because you didn't sleep well the night before or you're just not feeling like it. See the difference?

Tip 3—Give it time, lots of time.

It's so easy to say it isn't working. Just like the penny doubling every day, the results from your efforts take time to manifest. It does seem like results don't match effort in the beginning, but over time, the results are tremendous. Time is the secret ingredient. It is working.

Tip 4—Don't give up.

The only difference between those who succeed in anything and those who fail is that those who fail give up. For this to make sense, let's define failure. Failure is a lack of success, long-term success. Sometimes things work out easily, the first time. Isn't it awesome when that happens? But sometimes, many times, it isn't that easy. You have to tweak and try again. FAIL can be seen as an acronym: **F**irst **A**ttempt **I**n **L**earning. Ultimately, you only fail if you quit trying.

Tip 5—Pick one small change you can implement today in regards to your sleep.

Implement it NOW.

Tip 6—Pick one small change you can implement today in regards to your exercise.

Implement it NOW.

Tip 7—Pick one small change you can implement today in regards to your diet.

Implement it NOW.

Tip 8—Pick one small change you can implement today in regards to your relationships.

Implement it NOW.

Tip 9—Pick one small change you can implement today in regards to your mindset.

Implement it NOW.

Tip 10—Master one new habit in each area.

Then when you are ready, add another, then another. Take time to define your core values and decide what you want your future self to look like. Then, look to your future self for advice and motivation, and let your core values guide you. Master progress over perfection. You don't have to be perfect. You do, however, need to consistently make more deposits than withdrawals. Be intentional and make sure the path you are on is the one you truly want to take.

Alternate Ending

I can't help but wonder if things could have been different for Bob and Carol. What if Bob would have said yes to the repeated invitations from Jake to join him on his early morning runs? What if Carol would have made a monthly date night a priority with Bob, as she saw Emma do? What if they had gotten into the routine of reading books instead of watching Netflix a few nights a week and began meal prepping instead of grabbing fast food multiple times per week? None of it seemed like it would have made that much of a difference at the time. But now looking back, I wonder. We'll never know for sure, but I do know that small, consistent, daily actions do build up over time to create huge results.

Thank you for reading this book all the way to the end. By reading a book like this we know you are someone who cares about your health and is trying to live your best life. If you found this book helpful, consider giving a copy to someone you care about. If you want to connect with us further, we invite you to check out our businesses:

Dr. Libby Wilson:

www.bestlifefunctionalmedicine.com

Libby works with health-conscious people who are trying their best to take care of themselves, but despite their effort aren't seeing the results they are hoping for.

Nate Long:

www.longroadcrossfit.com

Nate loves pushing others to help them reach their true potential.

In health,

Libby and Nate

ACKNOWLEDGMENTS

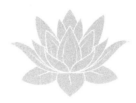

FROM LIBBY:

I'D LIKE TO THANK MY TOP FIVE FOR THEIR LOVE AND SUPPORT:

To my dad—for instilling in me a hard-work ethic and teaching me to always follow the rules.

To my mom—for teaching me to be fiercely independent and for working so hard herself to provide me with all she didn't have growing up.

To my husband, Andy—for believing in me more than I could ever believe in myself and for showing me that it's OK to break the rules sometimes. You bring out the best in me.

To my daughter Josie—for showing me what is possible when you combine the creativity and positivity of a dreamer with the work ethic, relentlessness, and drive of a realist. I can't wait to see what the future has in store for you.

To my daughter Ainsley—for reminding me to not sweat the small stuff and that it's all small stuff. I'm so grateful for your kind heart and your focus on the present moment.

I strive to be more like you all.

FROM NATE:

I'D LIKE TO THANK THE FOLLOWING PEOPLE FOR THEIR unwavering support:

To my wife, Crystal—your unwavering love and support no matter what crazy idea or dream I come up with is greater than any husband could ever ask for. Your patience with me and the support you provide our family is award worthy. I couldn't have asked for a better role model for our beautiful daughters.

To my father—the man that taught me how to work harder than anyone in the room, no matter if someone is watching or not. You taught me about what excellence is and that there are no such things as shortcuts in life. The example you set while growing up laid the foundation to who I am as an adult today, and I can't thank you enough for setting the standard and never wavering from it.

To my mother—you are the most selfless person I have ever met, a shining example of what a mother is truly supposed to be, and I am forever grateful for you stepping into our lives at such a young age. Your love and commitment to my brother and me is something that I can never thank you enough for. You're the best Maw Maw a couple of granddaughters could ever have.

To my amazing daughters, Madilyn and Marleigh—if there is anything I have done right in the world it is bring you two into it. Madilyn, you're an old soul whose inner beauty and determination makes me more proud every day. Marleigh, keep dancing to the beat of your own drum. Your loving and caring demeanor to all living things would make any parent proud. I couldn't be more proud of the two women you are becoming. Follow your heart and your dreams, and they will take you to amazing places.

To my brother—while it may have taken me 35 years to find my own path, I couldn't have asked for a better tour guide for the first 35 years of life. Without your direction I have no idea where I would be today. May our children have the same love and friendship with one another as we did growing up and still do to this day.

ABOUT THE AUTHORS

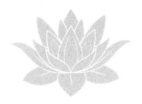

LIBBY WILSON, M.D., LOVES TO LEARN ALL THINGS ABOUT health and fitness and share it with others. Her passion lies in helping people achieve optimal health as naturally as possible. She believes strongly in identifying the root cause of illness. Her expertise lies in interpreting labs and designing supplement programs to help patients feel better, so they can then implement the necessary lifestyle changes to live a long, healthy, and meaningful life.

Dr. Libby is a board-certified family medicine doctor. She is also a certified IFM practitioner through the Institute of Functional Medicine and the Kalish Institute of Functional Medicine. In addition, she is a certified life coach through The Life Coach School. She is the owner of Best Life Functional

Medicine, where she helps people get to the root cause of their symptoms and fix them, so they can live their best life.

Dr. Libby resides in Springfield, Ohio, with her husband, Andy, two daughters, Josie and Ainsley, and their golden retriever, Zipper. In her free time, she loves running, CrossFit, reading, and writing. She thrives by coming up with challenges and taking small steps consistently to accomplish them. She considers her superpower to be consistency, which has helped her successfully complete medical school, two Ironman triathlons, over a dozen marathons (including Boston), and create her own dream functional medicine practice. Her passion is inspiring others to transform their lives too. To learn more about Dr. Libby or to contact her, go to www. bestlifefunctionalmedicine.com.

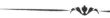

NATE LONG LOVES PUSHING OTHERS TO HELP THEM REACH THEIR true potential. This drive for continuous improvement has taken him on a less traditional path to where he is today. CrossFit was the catalyst that pushed him out of his comfort zone to get closer to his own true potential as an entrepreneur, leader, spouse, father, and friend. Nate's strengths and passion fall in helping people create systems in their lives to help them be successful in all five areas of health and wellness.

While Nate's formally earned a Bachelor in Business Administration and a Bachelor of Science in Middle Childhood Education, his most valuable education comes from reading the latest health and wellness books and integrating their various approaches. Nate holds his CrossFit L-2 certification and enjoys taking any specialty course to help teach people how to move better, sleep longer, eat healthier, be more mindful, and build quality, lasting relationships. Along with working with his wife to run two CrossFit gyms, Long Road CrossFit North and Long Road CrossFit South, Nate will soon earn his life and health coaching certification.

Nate resides in Urbana, Ohio, with his wife, Crystal, two daughters, Madilyn and Marleigh, and their two dogs, Toomey and Mocha. In his free time, he loves CrossFit, reading, traveling, and anything that includes enjoying new experiences with the people he loves. His passion is creating communities of people that love and support one another to reach their goals and true potential. To learn more about Nate or to contact him, go to www.longroadcrossfit.com.

AFTERWORD

Thank you for reading our book!

Love this book? Don't forget to leave a review!

Every review matters, and it matters a *lot!*

Head over to Amazon or wherever you purchased this book to leave an honest review for us.

We thank you endlessly and really appreciate your most valuable resource, your time! Thank you for taking the time to read this book and begin your journey to your best life.

Libby and Nate

NEXT STEPS

What now?

We, Libby and Nate, have read so many books that inspire us, but nothing really changes unless we decide to take action. As recovering taskmasters, our instinct is to move on to the next book and gather more information. However, our lives really change when we resist that urge and decide to take action. Download the free companion guide to get started taking action today at www.thepathofintention.com.

Also, we welcome you to connect with us on social media.

Join Dr. Libby's free Facebook group: Best Life Challenge. In this group, we take one small lifestyle change each month and implement it to move closer and closer to optimal health and an even more amazing life. Small, consistent actions build up over time to yield huge results.

Connect with Nate on Instagram at NLong23.

You've got this!

Made in the USA
Las Vegas, NV
28 December 2022